THE SAUNA AND COLD PLUNGE EXPERIENCE

A COMPREHENSIVE GUIDE TO DISCOVERING THE
PHYSICAL AND MENTAL BENEFITS, STEP-BY-STEP
INSTRUCTIONS TO BUILD YOUR OWN FINNISH
SAUNA AND COLD PLUNGE, AND EXPERT
RECOMMENDATIONS FOR ACHIEVING WELLNESS
THROUGH HEAT AND COLD THERAPIES

DAN BANACHOWSKI

CONTENTS

INTRODUCTION

I was on the brink of exhaustion, my body aching, mind foggy, and spirit drained. But when I immersed myself in the gentle warmth of a sauna followed by the invigorating chill of a cold plunge, I felt reborn. It was as if centuries of wisdom were whispering to me, healing me from the inside out.

Right now, you are going through a lot—and who can blame you? You might be feeling the overwhelming pangs of stress on your life from work, family issues, and much more. Compounded by health issues—never feeling like your body is healthy and happy—and the relentless pace of modern life, it might seem like you can never catch a break. I understand this as well as you do; life is a challenge, now more than ever, and this brings along the necessity of holistic, accessible wellness solutions that are not out of touch for people like you and I.

In search of solutions, here you stand. Maybe you are facing a yearning for natural health practices, ones that are much more stable for the body than ibuprofen chased by lurid 2 a.m. tap water. Perhaps you want to connect to ancient traditions, or maybe you just have an urgent need for self-care and rejuvenation. Whatever brought you here, rest assured that the solution awaits just ahead.

In this resource to sauna and cold plunge health experiences, you will gain a myriad of shortcuts that will help you understand these invaluable therapies and the role that they can have on your life. This book offers a comprehensive exploration of both physical and mental health benefits of sauna and cold plunge experiences. If you are looking for evidence-based solutions, you are in the right place. What's more is that this book offers practical guidance, including step-by-step instructions for developing your own DIY sauna and cold plunge experiences. You will also uncover expert recommendations for achieving wellness through hot and cold therapies that resonate with your goals through and through.

A bright future awaits you, one just like my current present. If you are ready to take this dive into enhanced physical health and clarity, as well as spiritual fulfillment, then why wait? All you have to do is turn the page.

1

THE SCIENCE BEHIND SAUNA
AND COLD PLUNGE THERAPY

E very day, thousands of people make their exodus to
the saunas, a simple yet fantastic endeavor that
serves as truly the ultimate escape from everything going
on in life. What's not to love about a sauna? They're social,
allowing you to connect with others. They also furnish
comfortable health benefits alongside their intrinsically
soothing and relaxing nature. Its equal, but opposite, twin,
the cold plunge, proves to be more than beneficial as well,
even if a little disarming at first. Did you know, however,
that saunas have a rich history that dates back thousands
upon thousands of years? It is amazing that they're still
popular today, and they are for good reason. Let's explore
what saunas and cold plunge therapy are to get started on
your journey.

A LOOK BACK IN TIME

What *is* a sauna? Saunas are a chamber of dry heat with relative humidity that can be used for various reasons. Typically, people enter saunas with the intention of merely relaxing, although others enjoy saunas for their health benefits. The typical sauna tends to be 158 °F to 212 °F (which comes out to 70 °C to 100 °C) in temperature (Sauna: Health Benefits, Risks, and Precautions, n.d.). Using a sauna can raise the temperature of the skin several degrees, inducing heavy sweating. This can also cause the heart to beat much faster in an attempt to cool the body. This is perfectly safe, though, as this occurs in a controlled environment and within a certain temperature.

There are several types of saunas; in Chapter 6, we'll talk about these types of saunas in more detail. For now, let's take a brief overview of some of the most common types of saunas you may encounter across your journey:

- Wood burning. A wood burning sauna uses wood to heat the room and sauna rocks. These types of saunas are typically high in temperature yet low in humidity.
- Electric heated. These types of saunas are high in temperature and low in humidity and employ an electrical heater that is attached to the floor to heat the room.

- Infrared room. Also known as far-infrared saunas, these employ special lamps to heat bodies, not rooms. The temperature is usually lower, but the same benefits can be attained.
- Steam room. These are not the same as saunas; they use steam heat with high humidity and moist heat yet achieve similar benefits.

There are also many possible health benefits that accompany regular sauna usage. These will be covered in more detail in Chapter 2, but just a portion of the benefits you can appreciate include less pain, lowered stress, improved heart health, and more.

Cold plunges are another method that are important and possible for you to encounter, especially in the comfort of your own home. So, what is cold plunging? Cold plunges are a part of cold water therapy which involve immersion of the body into cold water. This is often done in the hopes of obtaining a myriad of health benefits. People engage with cold plunge therapy both in and outdoors, and you can even buy and make cold plunge chambers for your own home.

When it comes to saunas and cold plunges alike, there is such a rich history that is well worth exploring. Across various cultures and for generations, both of these methods have been prevalent in health and healing. For instance, these therapies were used in places like Finland, Japan, and Native American cultures.

Believe it or not, the first saunas were developed closely after humans discovered fire. Fire led to saunas due to the impeccable connection that fire could be used to heat the body. In Africa, the first sauna was built. The original intention of these masterpieces was to rid the body of disease. In order to build these saunas, a grave-sized hole was dug in the ground. Then, a fire was placed in the hole. After turning to embers, poles were laid over the fire to create a bed that would then be laid upon—which rested approximately three feet above the fire.

After that came the Finnish sauna, which was utilized as early as 7000 BCE (Team, 2018). In Finland, a sauna is considered to be a necessity. At one point, babies in Finland were actually born in saunas, and even today they serve to play a valuable role in Finnish culture. It is also interesting to note how Roman and Greek bathhouses played a role in what we know as a modern spa. Designed as a social meeting place with the vocational intent to purify the body, bathhouses served as a striking intersection between a modern sauna and a modern swimming pool, believe it or not.

There are dozens of other cultures which birthed idiosyncratic traditions regarding sauna usage, and all of it is quite fascinating; so many cultures converged to grant us the modern sauna. But what about cold plunging? Does that have its own unique history? As it turns out, it does!

Beginning in Egypt thousands of years ago, the first cold plunges and ice baths were formulated in order to rid patients of skin irritation. Furthermore, the Greeks harnessed the powers of the cold plunge in correlation with an, at the time, innovative health module. Centering itself around liquids in the body called "humors," this health module proposed that cold plunges could actually benefit fevers and profuse bleeding. How impressive is that?

And what rings true to both of these therapeutic methods is the fact that both have been utilized over thousands of years. The health benefits—mental, spiritual, and physical—explain the popularity of these methods over the years, as well as how modern times have come to hold them as a beacon for health. Withstanding the test of time, sauna and cold plunge therapies are now even supported by modern science. Ancient wisdom knew far before we did that saunas and cold plunging could be so useful, and now this synergy validates the effectiveness of these practices. Do not worry; we'll talk about that in plenty of detail in subsequent chapters.

INTERESTING FACTS ABOUT THESE THERAPIES

Now, it is time for some fun facts about saunas and cold plunges. If you are interested in what you find below, some of the facts will be expounded upon in coming chapters, so fret not! Some of the most fascinating facts—

at least in my opinion—regarding saunas and cold plunges include:

- Using saunas can improve the health of your brain. This has been verified by multiple studies, even saying that as little as 20 minutes of sauna usage 3-4 times a week can be effective for lowering one's risk of dementia.
- Saunas can be beneficial for pain management. Our bodies release endorphins when they encounter high heat, which can produce an effect that lowers pain levels. This can work for anyone with mild to even severe pain.
- Saunas can improve sleep. Spending time in the heat, especially the controlled heat of a sauna, provides one with a mild tranquilizing effect that can be beneficial for getting enough rest at night.
- Saunas can improve the immune system and fight off illness. Exposure to heat and steam has been linked to higher white blood cell production, and those blood cells are responsible for helping us feel better.
- Between four and 10 degrees is the perfect temperature for an ice bath.
- An ice bath can reduce the heat felt by inflammation, especially after an injury.
- Much like saunas, ice baths can also help you get enough sleep at night.

As you can tell, both ice baths and saunas have the striking ability to provide us with a myriad of health benefits—and those benefits predate generations. But now that you have been introduced to some of the basics of sauna and cold plunge therapies, you might be wondering what exactly these methods can do for you, in more specific terms. That is where we're headed next.

2

THE HEALTH BENEFITS OF SAUNA THERAPY

D id you know that those who use a sauna four to seven times weekly were 63% less likely to experience death as a result of health problems and 50% less likely to die from cardiac disease than someone who rarely, if ever, uses a sauna (Sauna: Health Benefits, Risks, and Precautions, n.d.)? The health benefits associated with regular sauna usage are immeasurable, but to help you get acquainted with the benefits of saunas, we'll try to put those benefits into words. Let's uncover how saunas can provide you with stellar mental and physical health benefits.

PHYSICAL HEALTH BENEFITS

Saunas have so many health benefits that it can seem unreal. From heart health to pain relief and more, saunas can truly save the day when it comes to one's overall health. Let's explore those benefits together.

One of the most glaring benefits of regular sauna usage includes improved cardiovascular health. For example, there is significant research that suggests that cells, the nervous system, and arteries can be benefitted by experiencing saunas regularly (Andonian, 2022). It is true! And so is the statistic that you read at the beginning of this chapter. It was found that in Finland—perhaps one of the sauna capitals of our lifetime—cardiovascular health enjoyed significant improvements as a result of the country's regular sauna usage. And that is not just because they're Finnish!

Saunas are impeccable at improving heart health in many ways. For example, saunas can have benefits when it comes to those with heart disease. In the case of coronary heart disease, saunas can improve the flow of oxygen to the heart, alleviating some of the symptoms of such diseases. Saunas can even help reduce high blood pressure as a result of hypertension. There is also a marked benefit in the cholesterol profiles of those who regularly use saunas.

If you are not concerned with heart health, there are plenty of other health benefits to appreciate as well. For example, I mentioned earlier that saunas can lower one's overall risk of dementia. This is because the hot heat and steam has the striking ability to improve white blood cell counts as well as neural connections that benefit memory and cognition. Sauna usage can even help to improve some of the symptoms of dementia retroactively.

Furthermore, saunas can assist with benefits in the area of pain. This is because when you spend time around saunas, enjoying their warmth and steam, it releases endorphins into your bloodstream. Endorphins are responsible for pleasure and relaxation, similar to how you feel when you do something you enjoy that relaxes you. These endorphins can relieve pain by relaxing you, ridding you of any subsidiary tension that may be lingering inside of your body. This can help with your pain levels even if you are not feeling pain due to tension! Muscle strain and more can be remedied through the use of saunas too.

Similarly, range of motion can be improved with the use of saunas. This is similarly due to the relaxing effect that can be appreciated. Even if you suffer from chronic pain or similar disorders like arthritis, fibromyalgia, and more, saunas can be particularly beneficial. Between the white blood cell benefits and muscle relaxation, it is no surprise that these benefits are present.

It has also been noted that COPD and asthma, both severe and chronic breathing issues, can be improved through interaction with saunas. This is because when the hot steam enters the lungs, it can provide healing effects for these disorders. Although, if you do have COPD or asthma, you should definitely seek professional guidance before doing so—it is not for everyone.

Saunas can benefit those who have psoriasis and other skin conditions as well. As you know, steam is the result of heating up water until it becomes vapor. This paired with the severe level of sweating involved in sauna participation has been linked to decreased skin problems. For instance, the skin scales often associated with psoriasis decreased when introduced to a sauna environment over time.

Inflammation and cortisol can also be positively impacted by sauna usage. The steam and heat from it can prove beneficial for reducing swelling, especially swelling that correlates with an injury. Furthermore, saunas have been linked to a decreased level of cortisol—the stress hormone—in the body. This can also have significant benefits with regard to weight loss if you are struggling with stress-related weight gain.

In addition, toxins and heavy metals can be reduced in the body as a result of saunas. Sweating is known to release toxins in the body first, including separating ones from the skin that we absorb from pollution, bad habits, and more. Plus, trace amounts of heavy metals that we consume or are exposed to can be removed through sauna use as well.

Finally, saunas have been linked to the contraction of fewer colds and viral illnesses in those who frequent them. This is, again, due to the fact that saunas raise white blood cell counts and boost the immune system in response to the intense heat. As you can tell, there are dozens of physical health benefits to regularly visiting a sauna, and the benefits do not even end there; there are also plenty of mental health benefits to be appreciated.

MENTAL HEALTH BENEFITS

For generations, people have visited saunas for more than just the physical health benefits that they offer. There are also mental health and even spiritual health benefits that can be enjoyed as a result of regularly visiting a sauna. Understanding these benefits, in addition to the afore-mentioned physical health benefits, can help you understand your goals and personal values in sauna experiences —as well as cold plunges. Let's discuss some of the stellar mental health benefits that coincide with using a sauna.

First, saunas are amazing for mood and depression. A striking number of adults deal with depression on a daily basis. Who knew that something as simple as visiting a sauna a few times a week could make a difference? Studies have indicated that saunas have the ability to cause euphoria in those who go; this is the result of the stress that the extreme heat puts on your body (13 Proven Ways Saunas Can Improve Your Mental Health, n.d.). As a result, the body releases more of those endorphins we talked about earlier. And the better news is that studies have also indicated that this change in brain chemistry can become semi-permanent. Thus, we can conclude that if you visit a sauna regularly, you will be happier in the long run. Isn't that nice?

Another mental health benefit of saunas is that they can reduce both stress and anxiety. This is because saunas can, as I mentioned earlier, help control cortisol—the hormone that is responsible for stress. But that is not all; research has also concluded that saunas can decrease anxiety in many forms by increasing relaxation and decreasing feelings of frustration and anxiety overall. This means that dedicating a few times a week to sauna usage can also lower your likelihood of feeling anxious. Again, the effects have been found to be semi-permanent.

Saunas can also increase something referred to as "brain-derived neurotrophic factor," also known as BDNF. BDNF is a protein that is found naturally within your brain, and it serves the primary function of lowering risk of mental illness while boosting mood. BDNF does this by helping to repair cells, which often grants it the title of a natural antidepressant. Many researchers have linked low BDNF to depression and other mental health disorders. Some good news is that you can boost the levels of BDNF in your brain, and the even better news is that you can do so through sauna visits! This means that if you are worried about your mental health, you can preemptively help yourself out with a relaxing sauna trip!

Also, saunas increase the levels of norepinephrine in the brain. This one requires a little bit of background to grasp, so let me explain. In those who have attention deficit hyperactivity disorder (ADHD), it is common for the hormone and neurotransmitter norepinephrine to be lacking. This hormone often helps with attention and focus, and if you know anything about ADHD, then it makes perfect sense how a lowered level of this hormone can lead to attention problems. So, how do saunas tie into this? For starters, one woman who hit the sauna twice a week for just 20 minutes experienced an 86% increase in her norepinephrine levels (13 Proven Ways Saunas Can Improve Your Mental Health, n.d.). That is crazy; she experienced both lasting and significant benefits to attention and focus just from a sauna visit. This means that saunas may have the potential to do wonders for those who struggle with ADHD.

Myelin growth is also connected to the use of saunas. What in the world is myelin, though? Simply put, myelin is a fatty substance that coats or sheaths the nerve cells. Myelin directly allows for your cells to send messages both quickly and effectively, which is a good thing because it allows for the optimal functioning of your nervous system. Saunas come into play because the bodily stress promoted by heat in turn promotes the development of prolactin, the hormone responsible for promoting the development of myelin. This means that saunas can even help your nervous system work better!

We cannot forget the glaring benefit that saunas are able to help prevent dementia. Dementia is a major concern in modern times, as it represents the third leading cause of death in the United States. There is no cure, which is why prevention is so essential. An interesting Finnish study that took place over 20 years indicated that those who used saunas frequently were 66% less likely to develop dementia than those who rarely used them. In other words, a few trips to the sauna a week can help you lower your risk of dementia, which seems well worth the trip to me!

And I'm not done yet; there are so many more mental health benefits of frequent sauna usage, including:

- Lowered psychological symptoms of anorexia. Anorexia is an eating disorder where individuals fear eating or gaining weight, and sweating has had positive impacts on anorexia. This means that if you struggle with eating habits, saunas can be a possible solution to prevent your circumstances from worsening.
- Reduced chronic fatigue. Chronic fatigue is complicated, and it has innumerable symptoms, ranging from pain to sleep issues and poor immune system. Recent studies have concluded that the use of infrared saunas can reduce chronic fatigue as well as the associated symptoms.

- Reduction in tension headaches. Tension headaches can be detrimental to one's lifestyle, especially if they are chronic; however, studies show that sauna use can reduce the intensity of these headaches.
- Better sleep. Sleeping enough and with good quality is of the essence; without proper sleep, your mental and physical health alike suffer. The fortunate news is that saunas can help maximize the quality of your sleep, resulting in deeper and more restful, well, rest!
- Support of the thyroid. It is well known that thyroid problems can disturb one's mental health. Halogens, substances often found in tap water, can damage the thyroid due to the fact that the thyroid cannot differentiate them from the iodine it needs. Saunas can help excrete these halogens that lead to thyroid dysfunction and, thus, increased mental health issues.

Saunas are truly something to marvel at; they have the potential to benefit our physical and mental health in ways that many other treatment and therapeutic options cannot. They're easy to obtain access to, making saunas a comfortable option for most people. Moreover, they can both alleviate symptoms of chronic illnesses—mental or physical—while stopping others in their tracks. What's not to love about the idea of a nice, hot day in the sauna?

THE BENEFITS OF SAUNAS FOR SPECIFIC CONDITIONS

Sauna therapies can actually be tailored to specific health conditions. In other words, you can use sauna therapy to benefit specific issues that you experience with your health. This means that those with chronic health conditions, skin conditions, and more can benefit from the use of a sauna. However, it is essential to approach these therapies with caution and consult with a healthcare provider before incorporating them into a treatment plan.

Arthritis Treatment

One of the many chronic health issues that can be defeated through the power of a sauna is arthritis. Contrary to popular belief, arthritis can happen to anyone at any age—even children! Arthritis involves the inflammation of muscles, joints, tendons, and other components of the body. This can often result in pain, stiffness, swelling, and other issues that affect mobility and overall quality of life. Fortunately, saunas have been tied to improvements when it comes to the symptoms of arthritis, making it a compelling treatment option for those who can't or don't want to use other treatment types.

One benefit that sauna usage can have for arthritis involves reducing the stiffness of joints. One major treatment option for arthritis that people take advantage of is the application of heat to specific parts of the body, such as in the form of heating pads or other compresses. However, for most people, the relief is only temporary. This is where employing a sauna to your benefit comes in handy, as the effects of a sauna are usually more holistic and long-lasting, especially the more you use the sauna. The heat has the same remarkable ability to release tension in the joints, which can relieve pain and stiffness all the while.

In addition, saunas can improve blood circulation. Due to the fact that saunas open up the veins and arteries, more blood can flow to the other limbs in the body. In return, not only can the body regulate temperature more effectively, but the nutrients in your body can spread to other parts of it. This includes some of the areas commonly affected by arthritic pain. As a result, waste is also removed from these areas, creating an overall net positive health benefit. How amazing is that?

There is a third major way that saunas can help to relieve symptoms of arthritis. This benefit is pain relief. Heat is known to provide pain relief benefits, especially when it comes to symptoms of arthritis and other related injuries. Oftentimes this pain relief is not permanent, as nothing can truly "cure" arthritis; however, the pain relief is often immense and noticeable.

When it comes to treating arthritis with the power of sauna therapy, there are a few safety precautions to keep in mind; failure to do so can actually mitigate some of the benefits of a sauna. For example, those with arthritis should be sure to keep the temperature of the sauna to a moderate degree, especially at first. This can prevent dehydration and overheating. In addition, you should limit the amount of time that you spend in the sauna. This is a typical health precaution, and it can also help prevent excess pressure from being put on your joints due to heat. Furthermore, it is important to stay hydrated and always consult your doctor to ensure that this is a good addition to your healthcare plan.

Respiratory Issue Treatment

Another aspect of health that saunas can serve to improve includes the treatment of respiratory issues. Respiratory issues come in many shapes and forms, including conditions like chronic obstructive pulmonary disease, commonly abbreviated as COPD. While this can be a valuable tool for treating certain respiratory ailments, you should always talk to your doctor before using a sauna if you have issues with breathing. The extreme temperatures within a sauna can make it even harder to breathe, which can prove to be hazardous if not done with medical caution.

So, how exactly can a sauna provide one with respiratory health benefits? One manner in which saunas can help with respiratory conditions is through improving lung function. When you find your way inside of a sauna, you breathe in heated air, or in some cases steam if your sauna is in the form of a steam room. This heat can have striking benefits for your respiratory system. Mainly, this is because the heat and steam have the uncanny ability to relax the airways within your lungs, which proves beneficial for allowing you to breathe in more air and retain the benefits of such breathing. For many individuals with varying lung conditions, this can make the process of breathing much easier.

Another advantage that saunas can have on respiratory health includes the temporary reduction of respiratory symptoms. "Respiratory symptoms" is a term that refers to the combined symptoms often associated with respiratory issues and difficulties with breathing. This can include symptoms like congestion, coughing, and wheezing, which all have been indicated to reduce in the face of sauna usage. Similar to the lung benefits mentioned earlier, this is because heat can expand the airways and clear blockages. Additionally, heat improves circulation, which means that more nutrients are transported in, and waste is transported out.

Of course, using a sauna when you have respiratory issues isn't always going to be safe. If you have respiratory issues that prevent physical activity, for example, you should always speak with a medical professional prior to engaging with a sauna. Similar to exercise, the heat and temperature significance of a sauna can put excess pressure on the lungs, in some cases making it harder to breathe. If you've been cleared to use a sauna by a licensed medical professional, I recommend going for a more moderate sauna temperature. This can further ensure that you don't place too much strain upon your lungs during your sauna experience.

Skin Condition Treatment

The final benefit that I want to discuss when it comes to the treatment of specific conditions using saunas involves skin conditions. Many individuals suffer from skin conditions, even if they don't know it! Skin conditions like eczema, psoriasis, and even just plain old dry skin can be treated with sauna therapy as well. If you think that your skin could use some improvement, this might be a stellar option for you.

One of the ways that saunas can improve the trajectory of a skin condition is through improved blood circulation. As mentioned earlier (and as will be detailed more later on), saunas are able to improve blood circulation by expanding the blood passageways in our bodies. This allows blood to flow more freely from one location to another, and strikingly, this has benefits for skin conditions as well. A lot of skin conditions tend to be due to a lack of two crucial components: Nutrients and oxygen. When your blood circulation improves, both more nutrients and more oxygen make their way around the body, which includes the skin. This is how improved blood flow due to sauna usage can help your skin.

In addition, saunas have been linked to stress reduction by many. If you experience stress-related breakouts or flare ups in your skin condition, then you might particularly appreciate this benefit. Saunas allow the stress in our bodies to melt away, and that is more than just due to metaphor. When you expose your body to adverse conditions, including the abnormally high heat of a sauna, it prompts your brain and body to produce endorphins. Endorphins help us feel pleasure, and they're released to aid in the prevention of pain (which the body assumes is connected to the stress of the heat). This makes us feel less stressed, which can actually benefit the skin!

One important consideration to bear in mind before you enter the sauna to help with a skin condition is that your skin should be clean. This means that your skin should be free of makeup, perfumes, and lotions unless otherwise directed by a doctor. Otherwise, the heat can further provoke the worsening of your skin condition. Likewise, use moderate temperatures within the sauna to avoid excessive sweating, as the toxins released through sweat can exacerbate symptoms of a skin condition as well.

Clearly, saunas have the ability to help with the treatment of certain serious or chronic conditions, which is quite impressive! In order to achieve these benefits in the safest way possible, ensuring that your doctor thinks it is a good idea is of the essence prior to proceeding.

How Heat Works
in a Finnish Sauna:

The following diagram depicts the different heat zones you will find
in your sauna, as well as the way the heat moves inside it.

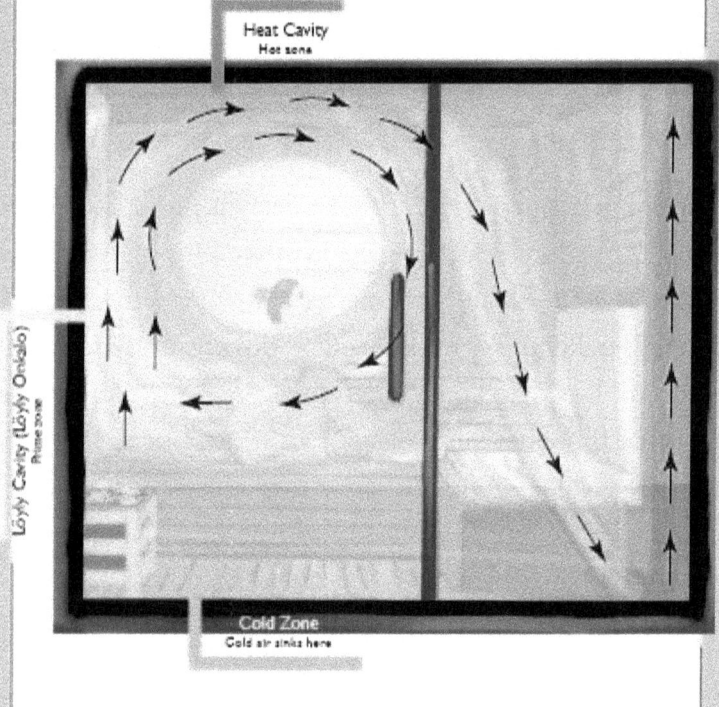

INVESTING IN SAUNA THERAPY: WORTH IT?

So, here's the big question: Is investing in at-home sauna therapy worth the associated time, money, and trouble? The answer will be unfolded in this illuminating section. If you are looking for the answer, short and sweet, here it is: Investing in a sauna for your home is totally worth it, and there are many reasons for that. If you are hoping for a more detailed answer, let's get going with just why this investment is truly worthwhile.

On one hand, the investment of an in-home sauna is worth it from a health perspective alone. There are dozens, if not hundreds, of benefits from having a sauna accessible in your own home, making a compelling case for the investment if you are truly dedicated to your health. Steaming up your bathroom with a shower is not going to achieve the same benefits as a dedicated, controlled area made to mimic some of the more professional grade saunas used to improve health. This is why getting an in-home sauna is, from a health perspective, more than worth it.

But it is also worth it from a financial perspective as well. An in-home sauna can be costly upfront, sure. However, did you know that owning an in-home sauna actually drastically increases the overall value of your property? This means that when it comes to reselling your home or other financial involvements with your property, you are at a significant advantage. I mean, in-home saunas are not all that common (yet) despite the fact that they are desirable. You can resell your home for an even greater profit if you take advantage of installing a sauna, and you get the added benefit of using the sauna while you live there.

In addition, there's a convenience factor that cannot be overlooked. Most health benefits accompany using a sauna four to seven times a week, which can mean going to a sauna every single day. Between going to work, actually working, school, raising a family, and squeezing in that much needed self-care time, the commute and time spent within a sauna can be out of reach. That is one of the reasons why the cost is well worth it to get an in-home sauna; you do not have to go far to appreciate the benefits.

Lastly, an in-home sauna is worth the cost because it is inherently a low-maintenance addition to your home. If your sauna is installed correctly, you just have to wipe everything down occasionally to avoid damaging the sauna, and you are done! It is much easier to own and maintain a sauna than it is to travel to one every day.

An in-home sauna is the perfect blend of health and quality self-care time if you are looking to appreciate the dozens of benefits that there are to regular usage of a sauna. But with all of this intrigue about saunas, you might be wondering how cold plunges play into it. Do not worry; I've not forgotten them. Now, let's take a look at the health benefits of cold plunges.

3

THE HEALTH BENEFITS OF COLD PLUNGE THERAPY

S o, you are interested in cold plunging. Here's what it is like to take your very first dive into a cold plunge. You expect that it'd be easiest to just jump into the cold plunge rather than prolonging the experience by going slowly—and you are right. Jumping into the icy water, you feel every part of your body freeze and then instantly go cold. The amount of tension in your body is palpable, and you have never felt a cold like this in your life. After about a minute, things get better, but wow, was it not hectic? How can this experience possibly have so many health benefits?

As it turns out, the health benefits of cold plunging are numerous. It might be an uncomfortable experience when you first start, but over time, it becomes far easier to manage. Just like with saunas, there are plenty of mental and physical health benefits to enjoy, and you will uncover them all in the course of this chapter. Let's get started.

PHYSICAL HEALTH BENEFITS

Let's begin with the physical health benefits of engaging with cold plunges. You might think that cold plunges are not healthy; dipping yourself into cold water cannot be the best for you, can it? But it actually can be!

One benefit of cold plunges is that they can enhance the recovery process due to exercise. Many athletes and casual fitness lovers alike use cold water to recover from intense exercise. There are a few different advantages to using cold water for athletic recovery. It can delay the muscle soreness that accompanies exercise. Studies have indicated that compared to other forms of intervention, or even no intervention at all, cold water has been particularly effective at slowing the muscle soreness, just to name one example. Taking advantage of cold water therapy after every workout, however, can slow muscle gains, so it is a good idea to use this method in moderation.

Cold plunges are also notorious for reducing levels of pain. Cold water has been noted to help with both short-term and long-term pain levels over time. One way that pain can be reduced by cold water is through the lowering of inflammation. Inflammation can cause pain through swelling, heating, and more, which means that reducing inflammation can lower pain. Contrast water therapy can also be helpful, which involves switching between hot and cold water. This has been used as a treatment method for arthritis and other forms of pain, which is thought to work by emphasizing blood flow. Finally, cold plunge therapy can benefit pain by lowering nerve pain or blocking the nerve cells that signal pain to the brain.

Furthermore, cold plunges are also particularly useful for improving circulation. Cold water contrast, as I mentioned earlier, is particularly helpful for improving circulation and oxygen levels in the blood. The circulatory system appreciates benefits as well, which in turn leads to healthier muscles and organs.

These benefits may not seem as extensive as saunas are, but trust me, when combined with the power of saunas, it is definitely worthwhile to participate in both sauna and cold plunge usage. From recovery to overall physical health benefits to the organs, cold plunges are amazing for the body and its systems. But what about mental health? Let's find out.

MENTAL HEALTH BENEFITS

The mental health benefits of cold plunges are plentiful and worth taking the chance on a cold plunge as well. Not only are the benefits plentiful, but they're unique from the mental health benefits of saunas too, making the two methods perfect companions.

One mental health benefit associated with cold plunging is improved mood. Especially if you are in need of a quick boost in your mood, cold plunges are perfect. Bracing the frosty water can actually improve your dopamine levels by 250% (Potential Cold-Water Therapy and Ice Bath Benefits, n.d.). Dopamine is one of the many brain chemicals tied to pleasure, which means happiness and relaxation can accompany an ice bath. Dopamine, in turn, improves our overall mental state. Even just a 20-minute cold water bath 4-5 times a week can be massively helpful for mental health.

In addition, cold plunges can actually help you build resilience—and it is more than just metaphorical. Challenging yourself to endure the cold water of a cold plunge can help you learn to mentally cope with stress, which is a transferable skill for mental health purposes. Learning to handle mental and physical stress can allow you to be more resilient in other situations, which is excellent for improving overall mental health.

And on the subject of improving overall mental health, cold plunges have also been associated with lowering levels of anxiety and depression, two of the most prevalent mental health disorders. Cold baths have been indicated to improve these experiences as compared to those who do not engage with cold water therapy. Even cold showers can provoke similar mental health benefits.

And how are these benefits gained? Predominantly, these benefits are the result of how cold plunges impact your hormones. Cold plunges can impact hormone levels in the following ways:

- Increased testosterone levels. This helps promote higher levels of energy as well as muscle development and bone growth.
- Increased norepinephrine. This can be particularly useful when it comes to promoting energy, focus, memory, and mood.
- Increased endorphins. These are hormones responsible for naturally increasing happiness and lowering pain.
- Reduced cortisol. Cortisol is the stress hormone. An excess of it can lead to weight gain, among other conditions.

Based on this information, we can understand that cold plunges do more than just make us uncomfortably cold; they also provide tangible changes to the chemical balances in the brain and body which are responsible for how cold plunges can make us feel better.

THE BENEFITS OF COLD PLUNGING FOR SPECIFIC CONDITIONS

Just like with the usage of a sauna, specific conditions can be treated thanks to the cold therapy provided by a cold plunge as well. As usual, be sure that you work in moderation and consult your healthcare provider prior to including cold plunges into your treatment plan; you never know if cold plunging can actually be detrimental to your unique system. Specifically, however, cold plunging can be excellent for the treatment of respiratory issues and skin conditions.

Respiratory Issue Treatment

We already talked about how saunas can be beneficial for issues with the lungs and respiratory system, but did you know that cold plunges can be equally as beneficial? For those interested in contrast therapy—which we will discuss in depth later on—or for those who can't or don't want to use heat, this can be the perfect option to aid in recovery and healing from certain breathing-related conditions. But how does it work?

The primary way that cold plunging can help with respiratory issues is through something called "bronchial constriction." In other words, a lot of people suffer from bronchial constriction as a result of their respiratory issues; cold plunging can help with that. This is because, similar to heat, extreme levels of cold can prove beneficial for reducing inflammation, which is sort of what bronchial constriction is—it involves the narrowing of certain parts of the respiratory system. By shocking your system with the power of cold water, you can encourage those airways to open up, helping you breathe far easier.

Of course, you should make sure to start with water that isn't perfectly ice cold; starting too cold can shock your system in a medical sense, thus resulting in *negative* impacts.

Skin Condition Treatment

Cold water therapy can also benefit various skin conditions just like hot therapies can. Mainly, this is because cold water can have an anti-inflammatory effect. If you suffer from a skin condition that is primarily characterized by inflammation, then cold water can help. This is because cold water is known for its ability to constrict, which can reduce swelling that causes a number of skin conditions.

It's vital to remember that everyone responds to heat and cold therapies differently, and those responses can vary widely. What works well for one person may not be suitable for another, and these therapies should be considered complementary rather than primary treatments for the mentioned health conditions. Always consult with a healthcare provider who is knowledgeable about your specific condition to determine if sauna and cold plunge therapies are appropriate and to receive personalized recommendations for frequency, duration, and temperature settings. Additionally, be attentive to your body's signals and discontinue use if you experience any adverse effects or discomfort.

COLD PLUNGE VS. SAUNA: WHAT'S THE DIFFERENCE?

When I talk to others about the benefits of saunas and cold plunges, one of the common questions that I get asked is how the two are different. So that you do not have to ask me (or Google), let's take a glimpse at the polar differences between saunas and cold plunges. Read through this chart to help you understand some of the key differences:

Aspect	Sauna	Cold Plunge
Temperature	High temperature	Cold water
Benefits	• Promotes relaxation and stress reduction. • Improves circulation. • Induces sweating, which may aid in detoxification. • May temporarily relieve muscle tension and pain.	• Enhances recovery by reducing muscle inflammation. • Boosts alertness and energy levels. • Improves circulation. • Strengthens the immune system. • May help with pain relief.
Execution	Typically done in a heated room or chamber. You sit or lie down in the sauna and sweat for a set time (usually 10-20 minutes).	Involves submerging yourself in a cold-water bath or plunge pool for a brief period (typically 1-5 minutes). Ice baths or cold showers are common variations.
Health Considerations	May not be suitable for individuals with certain medical conditions, such as cardiovascular issues or respiratory problems. There's a risk of dehydration (drink plenty of water), and it is recommended to avoid alcohol and heavy meals before using the sauna.	Not recommended for people with heart conditions or hypertension. There's a risk of hypothermia if exposed to extremely cold water for too long. Gradual adaptation to cold is important to avoid shock.
Mental Effects	Calming and relaxing; may promote mindfulness and meditation.	Invigorating and awakening; can increase alertness and focus.

There are a lot of similarities between saunas and cold plunges, but there are also a lot of differences. Did you know, however, that you do not have to decide between the two? There are plenty of ways to combine the two methods, which is where we'll go next.

4

COMBINING SAUNA AND COLD PLUNGE: THE POWER OF CONTRAST THERAPY

Hot and cold—two polar opposites, and yet best friends when they combine. Now that you know about all of the benefits associated with both saunas and cold plunges, you might be wondering which one is best for you. To that I ask, why choose? You can have both, and this chapter is dedicated to helping you find out how. Let's uncover what you can do to combine saunas and cold plunges for the ultimate contrast therapy.

UNDERSTANDING CONTRAST THERAPY

For a few years now, contrast therapy has been trendy online. Many social media users have employed cold water baths in tandem with hot sauna treatments for various benefits. However, contrast therapy is way more than just a trend; it is a popular method with just as many health benefits as saunas and cold plunges have on their own.

So, what is a contrast bath? The most popular type of contrast therapy is the contrast bath, which is a form of therapy wherein one takes baths in hot and cold water alternately. Most commonly, contrast baths are used for treating things like edema, stiffness, muscle issues, and pain, and it is most commonly used among athletes. Now, a sauna is not a bath, but a lot of people will engage with contrast baths by taking a cold bath one day and a hot one the next. It makes sense, therefore, that saunas and cold plunges can be used alternately.

Scientifically backed and powered by over 2,000 years of history, contrast therapy can be used on the limbs or the entire body. This form of hydrotherapy scientifically works by dilating the blood vessels, which then helps with blood circulation. Most contrast baths follow the following steps:

1. Begin by submerging the relaxed limb in warm water at a temperature of 100°Ffor an initial duration of 10 minutes.
2. Subsequently, immerse the limb in cold water with a temperature of around 46°Ffor a period of one minute.
3. Afterward, immerse the limb in hot water for four minutes, alternating with a one-minute dip in cold water.

4. Repeat this alternating four-minute hot water and one-minute cold water immersion sequence three additional times.
5. Complete the entire procedure within a 30-minute timeframe.

When you have a sauna and the ability to cold plunge within your own home, you can DIY your own contrast therapy experience. But first, let's explore the science behind why this method is particularly effective in more detail.

THE SYNERGISTIC EFFECTS OF COMBINING SAUNA AND COLD PLUNGE

By now, it is probably abundantly clear to you that synergizing cold- and heat-based therapies can be immensely beneficial, but you might have a few questions. How exactly does this work, for example, and what benefits can be achieved through contrast therapy? All of this and more are about to be demystified for you!

Combining the experiences of saunas and cold plunges is nothing new; people have been using these methods of contrast therapy forever. When used in combination, there are numerous benefits to be aware of that extend far beyond the benefits that only one option can offer. While the effects of combining cold plunges with saunas for contrast therapy are still being studied, with more and more research coming forth all the time, we do know about a few benefits for sure:

- Improved blood flow. The temperature differences between a sauna and a cold plunge offer participants drastically improved blood flow. Our scientific evidence for this is simple; heat expands and cold contracts. This works when it comes to the blood vessels in your body as well. Spending time in a sauna can expand your blood vessels, whereas a cold plunge contracts them. This forces the body to pump blood at a much healthier rate.
- Faster recovery from sore muscles and muscle pain. This works similar to the blood flow principle and is primarily why so many athletes and fitness buffs take advantage of contrast therapy. Heat and cold have different benefits for muscles and pain. Rather than canceling each other out, these benefits can be stacked and combined through the art of contrast therapy.
- Skin benefits. Both hot and cold water are beneficial for the skin but in different ways. Much like with muscle recovery, both of these benefits can be harnessed simultaneously.

Most people who do not believe in contrast therapy hold that mindset because, typically, hot and cold cancel out to make lukewarm. Lukewarm water is not going to heal anything, which is true. However, that is not how contrast therapy works. By employing cold water and then hot water, you achieve the benefits of cold and then hot water. You do not cancel out the benefits; rather, you achieve two entirely different sets of benefits that have little to no bearing on each other in a negative way.

The body responds very differently to hot and cold stimuli. As a result, we have contrast therapy that so many people know and love today. Contrast therapy is truly an effective and powerful method that can heal the body in more ways than one. One particularly amazing thing about contrast therapy that I have not mentioned yet is just how simple it is to integrate within other forms of wellness practices. That is right, contrast therapy can be combined with several other wellness methods for holistic benefits. Let's find out how.

INTEGRATING CONTRAST THERAPY WITH OTHER WELLNESS PRACTICES

As mentioned, contrast therapy can be combined with several other methods of wellness for more holistic benefits. For example, saunas are one wellness method that works perfectly with yoga! A lot of people wonder whether it is best to visit a sauna before or after their yoga session. The answer is not quite as simple as a one-word solution; instead, it depends on what kind of yoga you prefer to do or are participating in on a given day. If you plan to do restorative yoga, for instance, your sauna visit might be a wonderful warmup for the session (3 Benefits of Sauna to Improve Your Yoga Practice, n.d.). On the other hand, rigorous or tough yoga might benefit best from sauna usage afterward, as this can help to re-energize your body.

There are some other lines of thought on that, however. In my opinion, it is usually best to always go to a sauna after a yoga session. With that being said, though, there are numerous pros and cons to using a sauna before a yoga session. For instance, it can be a good idea to hit the sauna before yoga because it:

- Stimulates the flow of blood as well as prevents muscle stiffness.
- Can help your joints move more freely in various positions.
- Prevent injuries before they even occur.
- Increase your metabolism and heart rate, meaning that you will get more from your workout.

However, using the sauna before a workout like yoga can put you at a disadvantage as well. You might suffer from heat stroke or dehydration if you spend too long in the sauna, or you might experience muscle fatigue.

To contrast, using a sauna after yoga exercises can be beneficial because it:

- Improves the soreness that you will feel the next day.
- Helps your muscles release waste for a healthier body.
- Promotes weight loss.
- Improves the recovery process.

With all of that being said, whether or not to use a sauna before a session, and if you should use it after, depends heavily on your particular goals for sauna usage. Be sure not to overdo it!

Contrast therapy is something that everyone can benefit from, but if you are an athlete, you are probably looking for more targeted information on the effects and benefits of such a practice. Fret not; this is where we're headed next!

5

THE SCIENCE OF HEAT AND COLD ADAPTATION AND THE USE FOR ATHLETES AND LIKE-MINDED PEOPLE

S aunas and cold plunges alike are particularly effective therapeutic methods for healing, recovery, and performance enhancement among athletes and similarly-minded people. For example, let's take a look at the story of Jeremy, an athlete who practices nearly every single day and prides himself on his smooth recovery and performance.

Jeremy's journey did not start off that way. He works out a lot and plays soccer for a state team. At first, he did not have the benefits of saunas or cold plunges to help him out. After his workouts, he would come home sore and in pain. He could not enjoy the fruits of his workouts and sports, nor could he even enjoy a simple day off due to how much pain he was in all of the time. His muscles were always tight and sore, and it never seemed like he made any improvements or progress even with the most effort he could put in. That is, until a friend recommended sauna and cold plunge therapy.

Hesitant to try it at first, Jeremy did not think it could do much. After all, he took hot showers; shouldn't that be enough benefit on its own? But Jeremy's friend would not let it go. He convinced Jeremy to visit a sauna with him after a workout, promising that he would not regret it. Jeremy agreed, letting his friend take him to experience a sauna for the first time in his life.

Needless to say, Jeremy was thrilled with the results. Almost immediately, Jeremy's levels of pain began to decrease. It is like he could feel the tightness and soreness in his aching muscles melt away. Overjoyed at the benefits, Jeremy asked his friend what else could be done to help with pain and benefit his athletic career. Naturally, his friend recommended contrast therapy and cold plunging intermittently with sauna usage. Jeremy was more than happy to try this, and it turns out that he was thrilled with those results as well.

Now, Jeremy makes use of both hot and cold therapies every day. He cannot be happier with the results; not only does he feel better, but his performance is so much better as well. It is like he became faster, stronger, and more motivated overnight, all thanks to something as simple as using a sauna.

The best part of this story? You can experience the same benefits that Jeremy did. Whether you are a professional sports player, a hobby athlete, or just someone who loves to workout, anyone who leads an active and athletic lifestyle has something to gain from engaging with saunas and cold plunge therapies. In order to truly appreciate something, however, you need to understand how it works. That is why we're going to take some time to focus on how sauna and cold plunge experiences can impact athletes and like-minded people on a scientific level. Let's dive in.

PHYSIOLOGICAL ADAPTATIONS OF HEAT AND COLD PRESSURE

As you spend time in a sauna or cold plunge, your body is going to be impacted. Most, if not all, of the impacts that heat and cold therapies can have on the body are beneficial; you only run the risk of getting injured if you allow yourself to become dehydrated or something similar. With that being said, in order to make the most out of your heat and cold pressure therapies, it is important to understand the physiological and biological manners in which those therapies impact the body. First, let's take a look at the benefits of heat, as you would experience within a sauna.

Physiological Impacts of Heat

When it comes to exposing the body to heat, there are both immediate and long-term benefits to be appreciated. These immediate and long-term benefits are a bit different from one another, yet both are desirable in the face of sauna usage. When your body steps into the sauna, let's understand what's happening. Imagine your body is like the engine of a car. Inside of a car, there are so many mechanisms that respond to heat in order to keep the car working in tip-top shape, despite the blaring sun or the pressure put on the system by driving. Your body works very similarly.

One of the immediate physiological impacts of heat exposure is sweating. This is one of the body's first lines of defense against overheating; as a result of heat exposure, your body uses internal moisture to keep the outside of your body cool. This happens because when your body is exposed to high levels of heat, your sweat glands release a thin, salty substance onto your skin—a substance which we know to be sweat. This can cool the body down as the sweat is evaporated from the heat, taking the sweat as a byproduct instead of further heating your body. In many ways, this sweating process is beneficial. Not only does it jumpstart other bodily processes, but it is through sweat that a significant number of toxins are removed from your body's system. In essence, not only does sweating keep you cool, but it keeps you healthy.

Another short-term, immediate impact of hopping into the sauna involves vasodilation. What on Earth does that mean? When vasodilation occurs in the body, it is a response to heat. This is the technical name for how your blood vessels expand, as mentioned earlier in the book. As the blood vessels expand, it allows for heat to exit the body through the skin, very similar to the process involved in sweating. This is much like how opening a window on a hot day allows heat to escape the home; your body is essentially opening its windows when it completes the vasodilation process.

Let's go back to our car analogy. Some cars adapt to hotter climates in order to become more fuel efficient and better functioning. Your body is, again, just like this! Over time, your body takes the impacts of regular sauna usage and adapts to the "hotter climate" it thinks that you live in, which brings along with it some awesome health benefits. For example, there are improvements to your sweat that are certainly desirable for any athlete. When you sweat, your body releases electrolytes. Electrolytes keep you hydrated, which is why sports drinks are so popular! As you sweat more and more, however, your body adapts and slowly begins to put out less of those electrolytes in your sweat. This vastly reduces the risk of dehydration you face both in a sauna and on the field.

In addition, with more heat exposure comes an increased heat tolerance. This is because your body can (and will) adjust to nearly any environment you put it in. This includes the sauna. As you spend more time with heat-based therapies, your body can tolerate the heat better. In return, this means that you do not have to worry about heat stroke or overheating as easily, which benefits you both in the sauna and as you navigate your athletic endeavors.

As you can see, exposing your body to the heat of a sauna is both beneficial in the short-term as well as the long-term. Your body will adapt to the heat and experience a myriad of benefits as a result, which can contribute to improved recovery and tolerance of distress during your athletic participation. How great is that? Now, let's take a look at what cold can do for your body!

Physiological Impacts of Cold

Much like heat can benefit your body in terms of both immediate and long-term impacts, cold can too. Now, I want you to imagine your body to be like a cozy house on a cold winter's day, snow whipping around your walls. That house is going to do everything that it can to warm itself up, which is exactly how your body will respond as well. This very act of trying to keep your body warm enough is going to be accompanied by various health benefits as well.

For starters, one of the immediate physiological impacts of interacting with the cold is shivering. Shivering is like sweat's twin in that it serves the same purpose—regulating body temperature—but in a different environment. Shivering is like your body's very own built-in heater; your muscles contract rapidly, which can help generate heat through friction. It is the exact same concept as rubbing your hands together to achieve heat through friction, except shivering is like a nice, miniature full-body workout. This engages all of your muscles for health benefits.

In addition, just like heat causes vasodilation, cold causes vasoconstriction. You can probably guess what this entails! During vasoconstriction, the body tries to keep itself warm. This is like when you close heating vents within a home in order to keep heat concentrated within the areas you truly need it. Vasoconstriction involves the blood vessels becoming tighter, which keeps blood from flowing to your extremities in order to keep you as warm as possible. In tandem with heat, this vascular motion can produce improved blood flow benefits as well.

There are also long-term benefits to appreciate that can be obtained from cold plunges. For example, much like your sweat becomes more efficient over time, so does your shivering! As you practice cold plunging more and more, eventually when you shiver, your body will be able to generate heat more efficiently. Likewise, you will also form an improved tolerance to cold, which will mean that you can cold plunge more without being uncomfortable or missing out on any of the benefits.

Clearly, there are several physiological adaptations that can result from regularly using a sauna, cold plunge, or both. These adaptations are particularly useful for athletes, as they equip the body to function at a more effi-cient rate. In turn, this allows for improvements in both performance and recovery. Now, let's talk about something you might not be too familiar with: Hormesis.

WHAT IS HORMESIS?

It is a question that, without fail, I am asked every time I mention the word, yet hormesis is actually a really important concept that every athlete should be familiar with. Truly, hormesis is the secret to unleashing full effectiveness in your athletic endeavors, including saunas and cold plunges! Envision that you are a superhero training under a strict regimen for battle; hormesis is going to be that regimen. The concept of hormesis suggests that through small yet stressful encounters that the body experiences, your body can actually build up resilience and become stronger!

In other words, hormesis follows the idea that introducing something slightly stressful to your body can actually help you build up tolerance, handling that stressor with better health. If you have ever seen individuals with allergies visit doctors to slowly introduce themselves to the allergen, then it is an awfully similar concept; over time, their body adapts to the allergen, and in many cases, the allergy goes away. Saunas and cold plunge therapy can do something very similar to the body.

Hot and cold are like the dynamic duo of your training program. Heat treatments like visiting a sauna or even just taking a warm bath involves exposing your body to heat, which, in turn, provides the body with a heat stress workout. Doing so impacts your body in a few ways. Primarily, heat treatments increase your core temperature, which carries out various effects. For example, it is due to the fact that this raises your core temperature that you sweat, and as mentioned, not only does sweat keep you cool, but it also releases toxins. In addition, heat treatments involve causing your blood vessels to expand, which encourages blood flow in order to cool you down (which is beneficial on its own). This counts as hormesis because it is a manageable stressor that allows your body to adapt in a healthy way.

On the other hand, cold therapy through cold plunges and similar methods is kind of like a post-workout cooldown. Like stretching after lifting weights, spending time in cold therapy can allow your body to adjust to adverse conditions in order to allow you to operate more effectively. Shivering and vasoconstriction, as mentioned in the last section, are both effective forms of hormesis that can help your body adapt to adversity.

Much like cross-training is beneficial because it works out different parts of your body for holistic benefit, hot and cold therapy through saunas and cold plunges is like cross-training for your physiology; it allows your body to adapt to different forms of adversity in different ways. Particularly, this is appealing for athletes and those who are like-minded, because those individuals engage in activities that are typically very trying on the body. By engaging with both hot and cold therapies for contrast therapy, as discussed in Chapter 4, the body can adapt to a diverse set of circumstances, from extreme heat to extreme cold and everything in between, making the muscles, organs, skin, and overall physiology better equipped to handle one's lifestyle.

To sum it up, hormesis states that by introducing your body to minor inconveniences, over time it will build up tolerance. Much like practicing weight lifting with increasingly heavy weights will build up your strength, employing the principle of hormesis to hot and cold ther-apies will benefit you by building up your physiology's strength. By understanding the role hormesis can play in your recovery and training, you equip yourself with an advantage that, surprisingly, many people are completely unaware of.

THE ATHLETIC EDGE: SAUNA AND COLD PLUNGE FOR PERFORMANCE

Whether you are a professional athlete or someone who associates fitness with fun, heat and cold therapies provided by saunas and cold plunges are valuable tools that can truly optimize your recovery and training alike. While hot and cold therapies are not magic beans that will sprout your health into something extraordinary, they do provide a myriad of tangible benefits that can both enhance your performance and your overall well-being.

For example, heat therapy from saunas poses several benefits on its own. For one, heat therapy is great for improving muscle flexibility. Especially if you apply heat to your muscles prior to a workout, it can make your muscles way more flexible, therefore allowing you to perform better in sports. Much like warming up the engine of a car on a winter morning, the heat from saunas has the ability to help your muscles be more pliable prior to a workout. Then, applying heat after a workout can alleviate tension and pain, enhancing the overall recovery process as well.

In addition, heat therapy from a sauna improves your blood flow by allowing your blood vessels to dilate. I've mentioned this before, but you might be wondering now why this is such an important component of sauna usage. One of the reasons that blood flow is so important is that that blood flow is necessary for your body to carry nutrients to different parts of your body. This means that your blood flow being more efficient allows your muscles and organs to receive enough of the vital nutrients that they need in order to function, boosting your health and recovery.

Finally, heat can be beneficial to athletes due to the striking ability that it has to relieve pain. This is not anything new; many athletes make use of heating pads and other sources of heat to relieve muscle and joint pain, and there's scientific backing for why this works. By applying heat to your body, especially after a workout, tension within your body is able to relax itself. In turn, this alleviates some of the pain that you may be healing. This impact is doubled by the fact that heat can speed up the recovery process.

In addition, cold therapy can have tangible and practical benefits for athletes as well. For instance, taking cold baths or engaging with cold plunge therapy can bring down swelling, especially after a rather strenuous work-out. It can be applied to isolated areas or the entire body and can reduce both the swelling of the blood vessels and tension in muscles. Moreover, this also helps with mini-mizing the damage to your tissues as a result of strenuous exercise.

Another benefit of cold plunge therapy involves pain management. Cold therapy has the ability to reduce nerve impulses, almost like they're freezing them (but they're not; it is perfectly safe)! As a result, pain can be numbed until the area of the body is able to heal and feel less pain. Particularly, this method is insanely effective for localized pain relief. In other words, if just one part or an isolated area of your body is in pain, cold compresses and cold therapy can be just the solution.

Lastly, cold therapy can aid in speeding up the recovery process. Cold is known to reduce pain, and it can also reduce tissue damage due to oxidative stress. In other words, cold is able to slow or stop certain processes responsible for pain and damage within the body. This can speed up the recovery process, resulting in less injuries or downtime between workouts.

Beyond all of that, there are also three main and particularly notable benefits to appreciate as a result of both heat and cold therapy. To sum them up briefly, by engaging with hot and cold therapies, you can experience:

- Improved performance. Just like baking a cake, where certain amounts of ingredients are necessary in order for the cake to come out perfect, your body needs to be treated in perfect combination for optimal performance. By fine-tuning your ability to perform in workouts, sports, and other physical endeavors, you can experience more success with your physical activity and overall lifestyle.
- Prevented injuries. While cold and hot therapies will not stop you from breaking a limb if you drop an anvil on it, they do add a much-needed layer of protection to your body. When you take proper care of your body, which can be attained through heat and cold therapies, you face less of a risk as a result of your exercise habits.
- Boosts in recovery. Personally, I think it is best to consider heat and cold therapies to be part of the warm-up or cool-down process. They're essential, much like stretching and remaining hydrated are. Due to the scientific physiological benefits of heat

and cold therapy, you can make sure that your recovery time is sped up without experiencing any negative health impacts.

Remember, while these therapies can be valuable, they're not a substitute for proper training, nutrition, and rest. They complement your overall fitness regimen. So, whether you are a weekend warrior or a dedicated athlete, consider integrating heat and cold therapies wisely to optimize your performance and well-being without making unrealistic promises. Overall, heat and cold therapy are the perfect idea for any athlete looking to take advantage of some of the aforementioned stellar benefits.

Understanding your physiology as an athlete is vital for many reasons. Your body adapts to the circumstances that you put it through, as understood by the principle of hormesis. Furthermore, both hot and cold therapies can have immediate and lasting impacts that are worth taking advantage of for athletes, and the practical applications of doing so are immense. You might be wondering how you can achieve these benefits with increased convenience, maybe even in the comfort of your own home. Well, whether you are an athlete or a couch potato, it is as simple as building your own Finnish sauna right inside your home. Let's see how you can achieve such a dream.

6

BUILDING YOUR OWN FINNISH SAUNA

I magine you get home from a long, hard day at work. You kick off your shoes, roll your shoulders, and ouch! The pain from straining your body all day is starting to settle in, and it is only bound to get worse. After such a challenging day, you cannot imagine how good it would feel to just sit back, relax, and enjoy your time off from work.

What if all you had to do was walk into your very own, authentic in-home sauna? And it does not stop there; imagine how pride would swell within you at the very notion of having built that sauna yourself; all of your hard work paying off with the most authentic, spa-ready sauna experience.

That is what this chapter centers itself around. Not only will you uncover everything you need to build your very own Finnish sauna, but it'll be right in your own home.

Never again will a long commute or exhaustion stop you from reaping the relaxing benefits of a Finnish sauna. And the best part? These instructions are fully authentic. Let's get started.

DIFFERENT TYPES OF SAUNAS

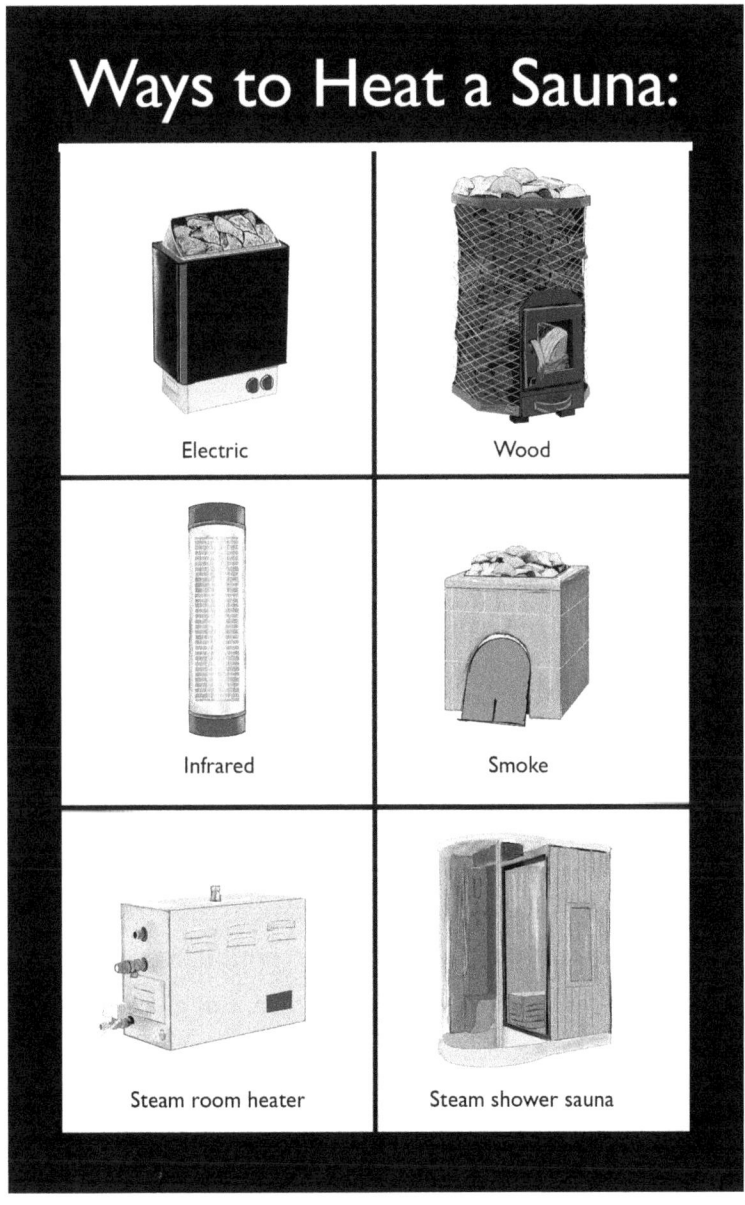

When it comes to building your very own in-home sauna, there are several different types of saunas that you will want to explore. Not all saunas are built equally; different saunas are built differently, of course, but they also use different heating methods, functions, benefits, and more. In this section, we will explore the six most common types of Finnish saunas in order to help you pick which one is the best for your needs. Let's find out which sauna is perfect for you and your home.

Electric Sauna

The electric sauna is probably the most common type of sauna used around the world. It uses something called an "electric sauna stove" to heat up rocks, and these rocks are able to retain heat in order to heat up the actual sauna itself. When it comes to an electric sauna, there's no need to burn wood as there is with other types of saunas. A simple press of a button can activate the stove for the sauna, triggering the heat. In order to create more heat, all you have to do is splash some water on the rocks. How cool is that? Electric saunas are often found in gyms and spas, but they're also particularly easy to install at home if you are looking for a really simple option. Smoke saunas and wood-burning saunas can be nice, but electric saunas have an advantage in that it is easier to control their temperature. If you are looking for an easy to build and use sauna, electric might be for you!

Wood Burning Sauna

A wood burning sauna, also called a "wood stove sauna," works as the name suggests; it involves burning wood. Wood burning saunas do have similar aspects to an electric sauna, but the setup is far more traditional. A metal stove called a *kiuas* in the Finnish language burns wood that heats up stones lying atop the stove. These stones then spread the heat to the sauna room. Water can be splashed upon the rocks with this method as well, which creates a steamy effect that most people recognize as the primary characteristic of the sauna. For obvious reasons, less people have wood burning saunas, although the experience is notably more authentic.

Smoke Sauna

A smoke sauna is the oldest and most traditional form of Finnish sauna, but despite that, they are not commonly seen anymore. Mostly, smoke saunas are the predominant form of sauna in Northern Europe, including Finland, of course. A smoke sauna works very similar to a wood burning sauna, but a smoke sauna lacks a chimney. Wood is burned in a stove in the sauna room, and the smoke goes into the room rather than out of the room or through piping. Once the sauna reaches a desirable temperature, the fire is put out. This does not impact the sauna's effectiveness, however, as they are built as a cabin with a design meant to retain heat. They are easy to build for a cabin, but it can take between six to eight hours to truly heat the sauna to the perfect temperature.

Infrared Sauna

Another popular form of Finnish sauna is the infrared sauna. Infrared saunas are a newer form of Finnish sauna that employ infrared waves to heat up the body. They utilize infrared energy, which is actually on a very similar wavelength to the energy we humans emit. Because of this, rather than heating up the entire room, infrared saunas have the ability to target just the bodies within them. This also means that the average temperature of the sauna room in an infrared sauna is usually much lower than the temperature of, for instance, wood burning saunas. Most people report enjoying traditional saunas more due to the fact that they provide a more authentic experience, but an infrared sauna will still grant you the same benefits.

Steam Saunas

When people think of saunas, they often think of steam saunas. Also called "steam rooms," steam saunas employ steam that is heated up and pushed into the room at regular intervals. Steam saunas in the United States and other major countries are found most often in gyms. Steam rooms usually work by heating up a steam generator; this generator boils water and continually releases it into the room. Much higher than the humidity of a normal sauna, steam rooms simultaneously manage to have a much lower temperature than other saunas. The humidity is what makes it feel so warm inside. This also means that steam saunas cannot be used for the same duration as traditional saunas.

One particular advantage of steam rooms is that they're usually far easier to clean than other forms of sauna; many other saunas have porous wood inside that must be deep cleaned, whereas steam saunas have tile that is far easier to wipe down. Steam rooms that are not made of tile are made of glass or plastic, which is similarly easy to clean. However, regular cleaning is strictly necessary for a steam room due to the fact that the moisture makes them more susceptible to mold than other forms of sauna.

Steam Shower Sauna

As the name would suggest, a steam shower sauna is like a cross between a steam room and a sauna. It is not a typical sauna, but because they're so popular, they're certainly worth mentioning. Steam shower saunas are also often easy to include in the home and are far more cost-effective than buying materials or labor to build an in-home sauna.

So, as you can tell, there are plenty of different choices available for your sauna-related needs. In this chapter, you will uncover how to build three of the most popular forms of sauna—a general Finnish sauna, infrared saunas, and the steam sauna. Feel free to find which one best suits your needs and get started!

STEP-BY-STEP GUIDE TO BUILDING A FINNISH SAUNA

Let's start with a traditional Finnish sauna. In order to build your Finnish sauna, you need to find a room or location for said sauna. Then, you have to make sure that the following room preparation requirements are met:

- Make sure that the heater cord is the correct model and in the right location for connection. Also make sure that it is long enough.
- Make sure that the cables for lighting are in the right place to be connected.
- Ensure that all of the walls and the lowered ceiling for the sauna are properly built and square, accurate to the necessary size of your sauna.

Then, you can begin. You're going to want to start with insulation and vapor sealing, which is completed by meeting these specifications:

- Make sure that the insulation boards are fixed to the walls and ceiling. They should be fitted against one another without any gaps between them.
- Where you have to fix the boards to studs, you can use screws; for masonry, use expanding foam adhesive. This allows your work to withstand temperature changes.

Then, follow these steps:

1. First, use general-purpose silicone to seal the lowest boards on the wall to the tiled floor. Imagine this like gluing them together to make sure there are no gaps at the bottom.
2. Next, you will need to drill holes for the ventilation ducting into the insulation boards, as shown in any drawings you have. Think of this like making holes in a piece of wood using a drill.
3. Pass the ducting through the wall from the inside to the outside. Make sure there's a suitable tail (a bit of extra ducting) left on the inside. It is like passing a wire through a hole in a wall but leaving some of it inside.
4. Seal the ducting into the wall using expanding foam adhesive. This is like using glue to secure the ducting in place.
5. Cut the ducting so that it is level with the surface of the insulation boards. Then, use self-adhesive aluminum tape to seal around the edge where the duct comes out of the insulation board. Imagine this like taping up the edges of a picture frame.
6. Lastly, use the self-adhesive aluminum tape to seal up any connections, holes, and screw-heads in the vapor barrier. Make sure to do this really well because it is essential for preventing condensation inside the walls.

The next part of the process involves working with the battens, which are what support the sauna benches. Ideally, your battens will be doubled up, meaning paired together, and the tops of them should reach 900mm and 450mm in height. As you fasten the battens, it is important to follow these rules:

- In places where you have to attach battens to the studs in the wall, it is necessary to use wood screws that are 80mm or longer.
- For spots where you need to fasten battens to masonry, first pilot drill, and then use 100mm concrete screws (or wall plugs and wood screws of the same length).
- Do not overtighten the screws—doing so can pull them through the vapor barrier, which is more delicate than you might think.
- Leave about 25mm of space between the battens and the corners of the room; this allows space for running wires and other hardware through the room with ease.

Now, it is time for pre-wiring, which is a really easy step. All you have to do is start running bench lighting and fan wiring, pulling the wires into the place they belong and taping them to the vapor barrier; this allows the ends to match with your wiring plan and keeps everything neat. Once you are done with that, it is time for cladding:

1. With paraffin oil, oil the faces of your cladding boards.
2. Drill holes into the cladding boards where you need to pass cables or wires through. You can actually do this while fixing them to the wall if you'd like to save time this way.
3. Use a saw to make cuts into the cladding; these cuts will serve as ventilation holes.
4. You're going to start cladding the ceiling. Then, clad the walls and drill the sauna ventilation through the cladding.

Next up, you have to deal with the benches. Oil the bench faces with the same paraffin oil that was used earlier. After that, you can screw the benches into place by screwing through the frame of the bend and cladding into the wall plates. You should install upper benches first, if you have any, and then you can move on to lighting.

Lighting is another super simple step to handle. The first thing that you are going to do is plug the end of the lighting into the plugs of the wiring you ran earlier, then clip the modules into the benches as well. Seal everything in place, and then get to work on the heater. For the heater, you are going to need to follow the instructions on the manufacturer's guide in order to install the heater. Then, you can connect it with the stones. Install your door, and you are done!

Top View of a Finnish Sauna:

The following diagram is an Example Layout depicting the components that make up a Finnish Sauna.

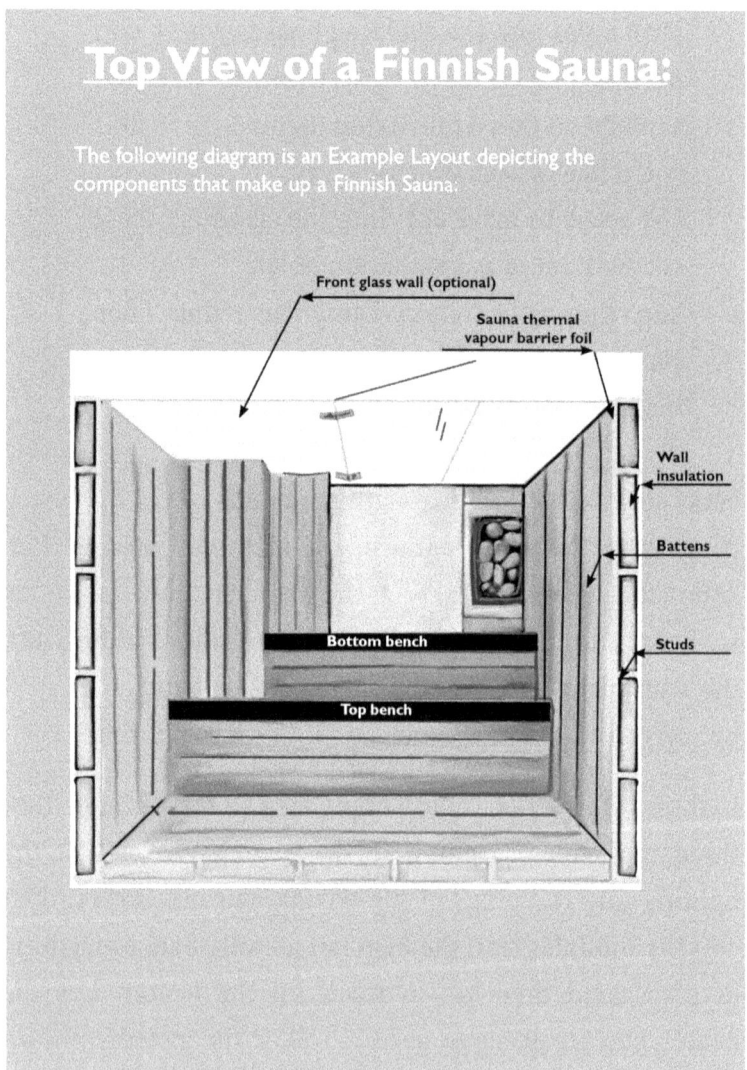

Front glass wall (optional)

Sauna thermal
vapour barrier foil

Wall
insulation

Battens

Studs

Bottom bench

Top bench

STEP-BY-STEP GUIDE TO BUILDING AN INFRARED SAUNA

Building an infrared sauna is, in my opinion, a much simpler process. The most difficult aspect of building your own sauna is all of the considerations that need to be made in order to meet your specific desires.

For example, the first thing that you will have to consider is the size of your ideal sauna. It can be tempting to get a bigger sauna—and I'll admit, they are nice and luxurious. However, you have to be honest about whether you truly have the space for a larger sauna before you buy everything you need to try to install one. One thing you should consider is the amount of space that you have available. It is also important to think about how many people you plan to have inside of the sauna at once, as well as if yoga or other activities will be performed inside of the sauna. If you are using a sauna alone and plan to just sit there, then a 1–2-person sauna is perfect. However, if your whole family plans to use the sauna, or if you plan to do exercise within the sauna, then a 4–5-person sauna might work better for your needs.

Another vital consideration for your sauna is the type of wood that you plan to use. Different wood for the construction of your sauna is not only going to appear differently, but it will have different benefits as well. For example, if you choose wood that heats up or contains sap, then your sauna will be more susceptible to damage.

This makes softer wood a more compelling choice for such a high temperature environment. Some of the best forms of wood for a sauna include basswood, spruce, and birch, as these woods are known to hold up well to the environment of a sauna. From there, it is up to you which wood you like the best!

The last step of the sauna building process—which is not really building, but it is still fun and worthwhile to consider nonetheless—involves accessories and amenity customization. Just a few customization options that you can consider include special lighting, smartphone controls, and more. While some of these amenities can add to the cost or difficulty of building your sauna, many people find them to be worthwhile due to aspects of convenience and aesthetic that are added.

Once you have considered all of the above, it is time to build! When it comes to infrared saunas, you have two options: You can completely build your sauna yourself, or you can buy an infrared sauna kit that comes with everything you need. If you opt to build your sauna from scratch, then you are going to need to measure your space. Make sure that you measure and keep in mind the fact that the inside of the sauna will be slightly smaller than the outside; you should measure with the outside shape of the sauna in mind.

After that, it is important to get the lumber, tools, and hardware necessary to build your sauna. You should make sure that the lumber you buy is cut to the exact size; if it is not, then your sauna will not work correctly and might let heat escape, both ruining its efficiency and potentially causing damage to your home as well. If you are struggling with the design of your sauna, you can find tutorials online that help you customize your sauna and meet your needs; even cross-reference a few different plans if you need to.

Something particularly advantageous about infrared saunas is that they come in pre-made kits. In my opinion, these pre-arranged kits are 100% easier to work with than building your sauna from scratch. If you are not looking for all of the stress and strain of building a sauna from scratch, an infrared sauna kit might be perfect for you. These kits will come with everything you need, and most of the time, they just plug into a wall. Simple, right?

STEP-BY-STEP GUIDE TO BUILDING A STEAM SAUNA

The final type of sauna that I want to walk you through building is a steam sauna. Steam saunas are quite a task to handle, but they're totally worth it if this is the type of sauna that you are interested in. Because steam saunas heavily employ water, you need to work with electricity and plumbing. This means that you might need contractors. You'll also potentially need zoning if you plan to build your sauna outside. Once you are ready to go, here are the steps for building your very own steam sauna.

1. Pick the location in which you want to build your steam sauna. As with an infrared sauna, you should make sure that you have the right size for your needs. Also, if you are planning to build a sauna outside, it should be in a protected area that is well sheltered from extreme weather conditions.

2. Next, it is important to plan thoroughly for your sauna. Again, you can visit blueprints online to help inspire you if you need to. There are various things that you should consider. For example, would you like your sauna to be a square, rectangle, or even some other shape? It is also important to think about seating arrangements, especially if your sauna is going to be used by more than one person at a time. Consider the materials and placement of heating and steam equipment as well.

3. The next thing that you need to do involves a bit of money. Purchase all necessary materials and tools, including lumber, insulation, vapor barriers, sauna benches, heating elements, steam generator, electrical wiring, and plumbing components. While these materials might seem like an investment, leaving any out or opting for lower quality materials to save money might result in a

lower-quality or non-functional sauna. Make sure to be wise with what you purchase.

4. Now, you have to build the frame and walls for the sauna. With the lumber you have selected, it is important to build a frame that is the right shape and perfectly level. Then, you need to install the vapor barriers and insulation that let the sauna retain heat and prevent moisture damage.

5. After that is complete, it is time to install the benches and flooring. You should build and/or install the benches inside of the sauna for best results, and then mount them according to your blueprint. Make sure that your materials are heat resistant and can tolerate humidity. The best flooring options are going to be cedar or tile.

6. The next step is to install electrical and lighting. I recommend hiring a licensed electrician for this part, especially if you have to install new outlets for the project. Get lighting with heat-resistant fixtures and make sure that there are places to plug in steam generators, sauna heaters, and lighting fixtures.

7. Follow the manufacturer's instructions to install the steam generator and heater. Ensure proper ventilation and safety measures are in place.

8. Install ventilation to control humidity and provide fresh air. Consider a vent near the ceiling to allow hot air to escape.

9. Finish the interior walls with sauna-grade wood, such as cedar or hemlock, for a traditional sauna appearance.

Then, you can enjoy your sauna! If you noticed, the process is quite similar to building a traditional Finnish sauna. If one instruction set confuses you, visit the other for improved assistance!

SAFETY CONSIDERATIONS

When it comes to building a sauna of your very own, there are a number of safety considerations to consider in order to keep you safe while building and using your sauna. Here are some safety considerations to keep in mind:

- For safety reasons, it is important to ensure that all sauna doors open outwards. This is going to help keep you safe in the event that you get trapped due to malfunction or other safety concerns. This is also the best safety practice for doors.
- You should make sure that your door cannot be locked or jammed accidentally. While it may seem like locking the sauna door for privacy is a good idea, if you pass out or otherwise become injured and need help, it is going to save your life to have the sauna door unlocked.

- Because saunas can become incredibly hot, it is important to ensure that there is no outward facing metal, such as hinges or screw heads, that one within a sauna can accidentally become burned on. For the same reason, it is important that the handle to the sauna be made of wood—a metal sauna door handle is going to scald you.
- All light fixtures should be appropriately fitted and certified for sauna usage by a proper electrician. You cannot use any old lighting in a steam sauna, as steam can cause damage to the wiring and possibly result in an electrical fire.
- Ventilation for the sauna should be installed properly and not covered by anything; failure to follow this requirement can also pose a significant risk of injury or harm to your life.
- The floor outside of the sauna should be non-slip. You should really trust me on this one; nothing's more un-relaxing than slipping on a hard floor after a sauna trip.
- If you have high blood pressure or heart problems, be sure to consult your doctor prior to using a sauna; saunas make your heart work harder than normal. Paired with certain health issues, sauna usage can be life-threatening. If you have high blood pressure, diabetes, heart disease, abnormal heart rhythm, angina or other conditions, consult your doctor.

- If you have just finished exercising, be sure to allow your heart rate to slow to a resting level before entering a sauna. As with the last point, saunas make your heart work harder; if your heart is already racing, you could face certain health risks.
- Wait to hit the sauna if you have recently consumed alcohol or recreational drugs. Again, overworking your heart can be dangerous. Furthermore, certain drugs and substances impair your ability to sweat or make it easier to overheat, which can be hazardous inside of a sauna.
- If you take medications that make you drowsy or impair your body's natural ability to regulate temperature, it may be best to avoid saunas altogether. At the very least, you should seek professional medical opinion before hitting the sauna if this is your situation.
- Using a sauna while pregnant can lead to dizziness, low blood pressure, and other health impacts. Be sure to consult with your doctor before hitting the sauna if you are pregnant, as you could put your own or your infant's life at risk.

Skipping safety procedures is one of the easiest things to do, but it is also one of the worst things you can do. You put your own life and the life of other people at risk if you ignore some of these safety tips, so do everyone a favor and make sure to follow them perfectly.

SAUNA ETIQUETTE

Before concluding this chapter, it is important to talk about sauna etiquette. The etiquette rules of a sauna are important, whether you are inviting others into your own sauna or visiting a public sauna due to not wanting to build your own. Sauna etiquette is vital to ensuring that everyone in the sauna can have an enjoyable experience and feel respected, which is duly important in a public sauna.

The first sauna tip that I have for you is to always shower before entering a sauna, especially a public one. Some public saunas have showers on site, but you should not expect it unless you have been there before. Showering beforehand is crucial for a few reasons. First, it gets perfumes and lotions that others may be allergic to off of your skin. In addition, it helps remove oils and dirt that can cause the sauna to get dirty. Moreover, showering prevents any smells or odors from emitting into the room because, while you are supposed to sweat, you are *not* supposed to stink.

It is also customary and polite to use a towel in the sauna. While you do not go in wearing clothes, you also should not go in completely naked; most saunas provide towels for you to use, and you should use them. There are a few reasons for this. First, it keeps a degree of privacy that is comfortable for those around you. It is also a good idea to use the towel because not only does this keep your bare skin from coming into contact with the wood—which can de-sanitize it—but it also keeps you from picking up germs that are already on the bench. Also, the seats in a sauna can be pretty hot anyway, so the towel is just an all-around good idea.

Another sauna etiquette tip is to respect the personal space of others. Sometimes, saunas get crowded; it is an inevitable aspect of using a public sauna. But just because the environment is crowded does not mean that you have to invade the space of others. Rather, it is a good idea to sit in a way that allows for plenty of space for others, not taking up more space than necessary unless the sauna is empty or nearly empty. This allows more people to use the sauna more comfortably. And while some of these etiquette tips might seem severe or strict, just remember that the etiquette rules and respect you show others are the same they'll show to you in return.

Also, while you are in a sauna, it is a good idea to keep the conversation to a moderate level. It might feel awkward to not talk in a sauna, just sitting around in a room with others silently. However, some people go into saunas to seek peace and tranquility. This means that, while conversation is welcomed in a sauna, you should be mindful of the noise level in the sauna and avoid harsh or offensive conversations inside. Do not trust that someone will speak up if they're uncomfortable because not everyone can do that as easily as you might be able to.

Limiting how long you spend in a public sauna is also a good etiquette rule, and a good rule in general, for a few reasons. Especially if this is your first time in a sauna, spending more than 15 to 20 minutes inside can be dangerous for your health. If you frequent the sauna, I recommend taking breaks every once in a while as well. Not only is this better for your health, but in a public sauna, there may be people waiting for space to open up. It might seem hard to give up your spot, but taking turns is what keeps the sauna enjoyable for everyone—plus, if you harm yourself in a sauna due to overuse, you will not achieve the benefits you desire.

Furthermore, when it comes to hydration, you should make sure to remain hydrated, but unless the facility you are at welcomes drinks inside the sauna, do not bring drinks, bottles, or cups inside. Not only can this cause spillage and damage the sauna, but drinks take up space that can be used by other living people. I mean, imagine if everyone brought a water bottle and set it down some-where; that is bound to take up at least a few desired seats. And nothing is going to embarrass you more than a plastic water bottle melting into the sauna and causing damage, so just save yourself the trouble and leave your drinks in the lobby.

Another part of sauna etiquette is to avoid allowing yourself to overheat. Not only is this a health rule, but it is an etiquette rule too. Overheating can be dangerous for you and other patrons as well. For example, if you faint from overheating, falling can hurt you and anyone you fall over onto. This can cause burns, pain, and overall discomfort that could have been avoided. Moreover, overheating and needing medical attention can disrupt the relaxation of others, so do not just sit in the sauna when you notice your body providing you with signals that say it is time to leave.

Remember how I mentioned that you should always use a towel? Well, you might be wondering what should go *under* the towel. There's no strict rule for this, as the rules for what goes under the towel depend on your facility. For example, some single-sex saunas allow full nudity, including the abandonment of a towel altogether. However, other saunas encourage swimsuits or underwear underneath the towel. What you wear under your towel is going to depend on facility rules, so be sure to find out ahead of time. But there are very few saunas, if any, that mandate complete nudity, so if you want to play it safe, wear a swimsuit underneath.

Of course, we also have to talk about cleaning up after yourself. Imagine going into a sauna and sitting down, and as you do, someone gets up to leave. When they stand up, they drop their towel, leaving the bench covered in sweat and leaving wrappers and a water bottle strewn about. Wouldn't that just sour your experience a bit? I know it would mine, which is why it is essential to clean up after yourself. Make sure that you take everything you brought in back out with you, including your towel. If you have left sweat on the bench, be sure to wipe it down before leaving.

Another rule that highly depends on your facility involves gender divisions. If you are in a sauna facility that has areas for males and females separately, respect that divide. People visiting a divided sauna are most comfortable with those conditions, and regardless of beliefs on gender, it is important to respect others and their comfort. As such, make sure that you visit the sauna area that matches your gender and avoid the opposite sauna to be respectful of the rules and the others visiting the sauna.

Lastly, it is important to silence your phone and be respectful while entering or exiting the sauna. No one wants to hear a ringtone from across the sauna. Moreover, it is important to make sure that when you leave the sauna, you do not want to let too much cold in as this can disturb others.

Sauna etiquette might seem like a lot of pointless rules that you do not want to follow but trust me; you do not want to feel uncomfortable in such a vulnerable place. By following these rules, not only do you respect others, but you ensure that they will respect you as well. If you notice a newbie breaking a rule, kindly let them know and make them feel comforted—most people do not intentionally go into saunas to be rude. Overall, the etiquette of saunas depends on your facility and is not universal, so make sure to understand the environment you are in as well.

Building your own sauna in your home does not have to be a challenge; with the information in this chapter, not only can you build your very own sauna in your home, but you can pick which sauna is best for you. Coupled with the right safety precautions, using a sauna that is on your very own property can be a life-changing experience in the best of ways. Isn't that amazing?

7

BUILDING YOUR OWN COLD PLUNGE

I n the last chapter, we focused on how you can build your own sauna. This takes so much of the challenge out of the experience; it allows you to enjoy the benefits of a sauna in your own home. What more could you ask for? Well, a cold plunge, of course! Cold plunges come with their own idiosyncratic benefits, as we discussed in previous chapters. Something a bit shocking about cold plunges, however, is that they're hard to come by in places like gyms or spas; instead, you are expected to take a cold shower, and that is not quite the same. The solution is simple! All you have to do is build your own cold plunge. Coupled with your own sauna, you have everything you need for contrast therapy in your own home. Now that is cool.

In this captivating chapter, you will master the art of building a cold plunge right in your own home. It is up to you if you also want a sauna—if you have the space, having both is certainly something that I recommend. Whichever way you decide to go, let's get started.

OPTIONS AND ESSENTIALS

When it comes to your own DIY cold plunge experience, you do not have to shell out tons of cash in order to get it. In fact, cold plunges can be cheap or even free, making a compelling case for having both a cold plunge and a sauna if you were going to have a sauna alone. There are also a multitude of options when it comes to building your own cold plunge, many of which require little-to-no space. Compared to a sauna, the experience of building your own cold plunge is a piece of cake. First, we're going to talk about the different cold plunge options that you have, as well as what you need for each one.

One of the most popular methods of DIY-ing a cold plunge at home is a cold plunge tub. A cold plunge tub is a comfortable, one-person cold plunge experience that is simple and cost effective. It allows you to submerge your body up to the neck in cold water and only needs a few materials. First, you'd need a large container or plastic storage bin. This container should be big enough to hold you, yet sturdy enough to hold the pressure of the water and other materials. You also need insulation. This is meant to keep the water cold, and you can use almost anything—

blankets, foam, and more are all common options. You'll probably need some ice if you want a true cold plunge experience. The only materials that you will need include a saw, drill, thermometer, and measuring tape.

Another option that you have is the cold plunge barrel, which is perfect for if you do not want to spend a lot on high quality materials—the quality of your materials matters significantly less when it comes to a cold plunge than a sauna. For this type of in-home cold plunge, you are going to need a large barrel, like one used for whisky or wine. You can get these from a few different places. You also need insulation and ice, as well as something like a pool liner. For this type of cold plunge, you might also opt for a drainage system; this way, you do not have to tip the barrel over every time you need to drain it. You'll need the same tools as last time as well.

Some people opt for a cold plunge pool instead, which is often a classier, yet high maintenance, alternative to the cold plunge barrel. Often laid out as an in or above ground pool, if you plan to spend lots of time cold plunging and wish to do so comfortably, this may be your option—especially if you have the money to spend. For this cold plunge, you are going to need quite a few things: A shovel, concrete blocks, concrete mix, waterproof liner, and a pump and filter. You also need a measuring tape, level, trowel, and rubber mallet to build with. More beautiful and permanent than a barrel cold plunge, I recommend cold plunge pools for anyone who thinks they might be the perfect addition to their home.

Did you know you can actually build a cold plunge from a chest freezer? It is true! Not everyone has the space or means to go for some of the aforementioned options, which is when many people choose to go for the cold plunge freezer option. It is smaller, discrete, and has built-in insulation. This means you just need the freezer, some PVC, and sealant. To personalize and install the cold plunge freezer, you may also need a drill, saw, sandpaper, tape measure, and more. It is a much easier process than it sounds like.

There are several other cold plunge alternatives that you might opt to take advantage of as well. These options include:

- Cold plunge chiller. This process involves buying or creating a chiller to cool down the water in a pre-existing pool or tub. If you already have a pool or even just have a bathtub, this may be a compelling option. It is an option that requires less building but more technical knowledge in order to employ, necessitating the water chiller unit itself and a few other tools. A basic toolkit should be sufficient, and it is important to use materials, space, and resources that will not degrade as a result of water exposure or cold exposure.

Otherwise, your cold plunge will not last very long.

- Cold plunge horse trough. Yes, you heard me right, a horse trough! You would not believe some of the things that people have access to, and if you have access to a horse trough, then you are in luck when it comes to cold plunging. This is also a good option for those looking to build a cold plunge that holds multiple people at a time. For this, you need a horse trough made from galvanized steel, a water pump, a filter, and pool chemicals if you plan to reuse the same water.

Overall, when it comes to organizing a cold plunge experience in the comfort of your own home—or backyard—it is relatively simple; with the right materials, a vision, and time, you can bring cold plunging to you, making it much more convenient to attain the health benefits we talked about earlier.

Before moving on to the instructional aspect of the chapter, I wanted to take a moment to talk about the usage of the freezer tub method. The outdoor freezer chest method has been used for decades, and it is actually a pretty successful method, which is why I wanted to mention it. Many people have touted it for its price; for only a couple hundred dollars, you can build a sizable, comfortable, and best of all, effective cold plunge that meets your specifications perfectly. Another benefit of cold plunge freezers is that they come insulated, which means that there is far less work involved in the making of your cold plunge. All of this is to say, if you do not feel like doing much, go for this option. Otherwise, let's see how you can build your own cold plunge tub or pool!

STEP-BY-STEP GUIDE TO BUILDING A COLD PLUNGE TUB OR POOL

So, you are interested in building your own cold plunge tub or pool. You got a brief overview earlier, but what now? Well, you get started with the building process, of course. This section is dedicated to helping you build your very own cold plunge tub or pool right at home. So, get ready, grab your tools, and let's get started.

Cold Plunge Tub Instructions

The first option that I'll walk you through is the cold plunge tub, which can be done with a plastic tub or even a wooden barrel. For this, you are going to need the following materials:

- A large container that can hold you and water
- Insulation
- Saw
- Drill
- Thermometer
- Measuring tape
- Ice (optional)

Once you have collected those items, it is time to get started. In order to build your very own cold plunge tub, follow these instructions:

1. Select your container. You do not have to use any specific kind of container, but it should be big enough for the biggest person cold plunging to fit inside. The walls should also be able to hold up to the weight of the water within them. Many people often opt for those large, cheap plastic storage bins, metal tubs, and even large metal trash cans for their needs.

2. Next, you are going to need to add insulation. Insulation is going to be what keeps the water inside of your tub cold—as long as that water was cold in the first place. For this type of cold plunge, most people opt for using hay bales, blankets, or foam for insulation. You're going to need to cut the insulation to fit the inside of the container, making sure that it covers the sides and the bottom. Then, use your materials to attach the insulation if needed.

3. Now, you can add water. Fill the container with cold water, adding ice now or during the next step.

4. Your cold plunge should be between 50 and 60 degrees for optimal results. Now, you should measure the temperature of your cold plunge

and see where it falls. If the temperature is too warm for your liking, you can add some ice now.

5. A drainage system for your cold plunge will allow you to easily change the water in your cold plunge without having to tip the whole thing over. You can do so by drilling a hole near the bottom of the cold plunge, and then attaching a valve or hose to that.

6. Use your cold plunge! Now, you can go ahead and get into your cold plunge. At first, it is going to be hard to spend more than a few minutes—or even a few seconds—in the cold plunge. Listen to your body and slowly increase the time you spend in the cold plunge, rather than forcing yourself to endure long periods of time at once.

For most people, this version of a cold plunge works perfectly. It allows people to make a quick and easy cold plunge that is just as effective as a big, fancy cold plunge method—like a cold plunge pool. And speaking of, if a cold plunge pool is your style, that is what we're going to build next.

Cold Plunge Pool Instructions

A cold plunge pool is a more permanent, high mainte-nance, yet classy, cold plunge method. If you plan to cold plunge socially, often, or even just with family, investing in the time and materials necessary to build a cold plunge pool can be purely spectacular. Here's what you need to build a cold plunge pool:

- Shovel
- Concrete blocks or bricks
- Concrete mix
- Waterproof liner
- Measuring tape
- Level
- Trowel
- Rubber mallet
- Pump and filter (optional)

Once you have gathered your materials, here are the instructions to follow:

1. Start off by planning where your pool is going to go and what size it will be. You should pick a space where the ground is flat and, obviously, there is enough space for your plans. Usually, plunge pools are about eight feet around and four feet deep, but you can resize to your needs.
2. Dig out the space in which you plan to build your plunge pool. Your hole needs to be at least six inches bigger than each measurement; for example, if you are going four feet deep, then you need to dig four and a half feet deep. Use your level to ensure that the bottom of the hole is as flat and as even as possible.

3. Next, you are going to build the pool wall. You're going to use your concrete bricks or blocks in order to create a wall that follows the perimeter (sides) of the pool. As you do, make sure the wall is level and flush against the inside of the hole.

4. Then, you need to follow the instructions on your concrete mix in order to pour the concrete in the right consistency. Use the trowel to spread the concrete out between the cracks in the wall and then let the concrete dry for at least a duration of 24 hours.

5. Once your concrete is dry, install the waterproof liner into the plunge pool. You should smooth it out to ensure that there are no wrinkles or air bubbles, and then cut the excess material to meet the edges of the pool.

6. If you have opted for a pump and filter, now is the time to install that as well. This will help keep your plunge pool water clean and sanitary. Your pump and filter will come with instructions; those are what you should follow for this step.

7. Finally, fill the pool with water and add ice to your desired temperature.

And tada! You're ready to enjoy your cold plunge pool.

SOME COLD PLUNGE TIPS

When you first start to cold plunge, you might have a lot of questions; you might be wondering how you can keep yourself safe, what you should or should not do, and more. Allow me to spend a few moments dispelling the confusion. When you first start cold plunging, some things that you *should* do include:

- Beginning with a lower water temperature. When you first start plunging, it might be tempting to crank the temperature down all the way right away. Do not do that; by doing so, you risk frostbite and physical injury. Instead, if you want to get the water down to 50°F to 60°F, start at a higher temperature and slowly lower it until you are comfortable in that range.
- Understanding your limits. Not everyone can handle the same temperature for the same duration. If 60-degree water is absolutely too much for you, then warm it up some; not only does this keep you safe, but because your body responds to this temperature the same as someone else might respond to a lower one, you still receive the benefits of the cold plunge. There's no shame in listening to your body about these things.
- Wearing clothes that help you maintain your body temperature. Hypothermia is no joke; you should always cold plunge in proper clothing to avoid

this and damage to your skin. This does not impact the benefits of a cold plunge; rather, it just keeps you safe.

- Making a schedule for when you engage with cold plunging. It can be time consuming to keep up with your cold plunge schedule, but it is worthwhile. By ensuring that you engage with cold plunging regularly, you can keep your tolerance to the cold up. It is also helpful in sustaining the benefits you experience long-term, as well as ensuring that the cold is not a shock to your system.

By keeping these cold plunge dos in mind, you can ensure that your experience is both positive and beneficial to your health. The best part is that these recommendations are not even that hard to include into your cold plunge routine! In addition, there are a handful of things that you should avoid doing when you cold plunge, which include:

- Not forcing your body to work harder than it is able to. Your body has physiological limits on what it can and cannot do, and you will understand where that limit is as you begin to cold plunge more and more. If you attempt to push your body beyond the comfortable limits of what it can handle, then you are sure to experience harm and even danger from the experience of cold plunging. This is so easy to prevent if you know how!

- Not staying in the cold plunge for too long. Believe it or not, six to eight minutes is all you need to experience spectacular benefits as a result of your cold plunge routine. You do not have to spend hours—or even just half of one—in the cold plunge. If you do force yourself to stay in for much longer, then you risk your health and safety as a result. That is not worth it at all! Keep your health safe by getting out when it is too much, and slowly increasing up to that six-minute goal if you would like.

- Not going in alone, especially at first. Some people are prone to fainting or passing out when they endure a dramatic shift in temperature. Instead of going in alone, it is always a good idea to have someone with you, whether they're actually plunging with you or not. It is a safety precaution that can preserve your life in a worst-case scenario.

- Not taking a hot or even warm bath after your ice bath. Contrast therapy is certainly effective, but you have to let your body come back up to its normal temperature before you try a sauna or even a bath. Otherwise, you can shock your body and potentially cause further health issues as a result. I recommend waiting a minimum of a half hour between your cold plunge and any heat therapy you plan to engage with for the best benefits, but even waiting a day or two can be helpful as well!

To keep you safe, it is crucial to avoid the above list of cold plunging do nots. Otherwise, you pose a risk to yourself in more ways than one, and no one wants to endure health issues when they try to experience health *benefits*. With all of this in mind, you have the ability to be a successful first-time cold plunger.

COLD PLUNGE ALTERNATIVES

After hearing about the building process, advantages, safety tips, and more pertaining to cold plunging, many people often wonder if there are alternative forms of cold therapy, as well as how those alternative options stand up to a cold plunge. As it turns out, there are a few different alternative options that you can take a look at when it comes to cold therapy.

First, let's go over the benefits and drawbacks that are often associated with cold plunges. One praise many people often sing to cold plunges is that they're so accessible. Just above you saw how easy it is to make your old cold plunge system, and beyond that, they're also accessible at plenty of gyms, spas, and other locations. This means that if you want to take a cold plunge, you don't usually have to go far. In addition, many people also appreciate the fact that you can control the temperature by adding ice. This is particularly beneficial because it means that a cold plunge is customizable; you can allow the temperature to be as cold (or even warm, if you're new) as you can stand. Finally, traditional cold plunges offer a full immersion benefit, wherein the entire body can be submerged. This provides more encompassing benefits and is a major pro for many individuals.

Despite this, there are a few drawbacks that can leave cold plunge enthusiasts in search of alternative methods. For example, building your own cold plunge in your home or yard is a spacious requirement; it involves having both enough space for the tub itself, but space for you to safely enter and exit as well. For individuals in apartments or other shared living settings, this is simply not possible. Beyond that, maintaining the water of a cold plunge can be tricky for some people. If you plan to reuse the water, cleaning and sanitizing the water between uses can be hard; if you don't, you still have to drain and refill the cold plunge each time. Not to mention that the cold plunge only sustains the ideal temperature for a few minutes at a time. Lastly, a common complaint that I hear from individuals regarding cold plunging is that they can't just sit inside and relax—due to the temperature, sessions have to be limited in duration.

The good news is that if you share some of these disdainful aspects with cold plungers, or if you're looking for more of a particular benefit, then there are plenty of options for you to take advantage of, most of which are easily accessible in some regard. These alternatives, while not cold plunges themselves, can be used to simulate similar benefits and achieve health advantages overall.

The first cold plunge alternative that you should know of is the cryotherapy chamber. This is exactly what it sounds like, and there are many benefits (and a few drawbacks) to the use of cryotherapy chambers. For example, a lot of people like that you only have to be inside for two to three minutes to experience the same benefits as a longer cold plunge session. This does wonders to reduce the discomfort often associated with the extreme temperature. In addition, many adore the available temperature controls. Because cryotherapy chambers don't use water and ice—instead opting for a liquid nitrogen cooling mechanism—it is simple to not only customize the chamber's temperature but to maintain that temperature as well. Moreover, these chambers also provide users with similar full body benefits to cold plunges, which has been associated with positive health benefits. This includes, just to name a few, improved circulation, inflammation, and muscle recovery.

On the flip side, there are some disadvantages to be aware of if you want to try out a cryotherapy chamber. One is the cost that is typically associated with cold chamber usage. Almost no one has an at-home cryotherapy chamber, and visiting a location with cryotherapy chambers can be a bit costly. This, compared to other methods that are cheap or even free, proves to be a significant disadvantage. Furthermore, a lot of people report having issues with finding these cryotherapy chambers in the first place. Due to spacial and cost requirements, cryotherapy chambers are mostly found in wellness centers and/or clinics. This can make them particularly hard to find, especially if you live in a smaller area. Then, some individuals who have used cryotherapy chambers have reported potential health risks, such as experiencing frostbite or other skin irritations. As these drawbacks can be potentially life threatening, always consult with your healthcare provider before hopping into one of these chambers.

Another alternative for cold plunge therapy is the good old cold shower. Many people adore cold showers as an alternative to cold plunges, and there are a few reasons for this. Chief among those reasons is convenience. Everyone who has access to a showerhead also has access to a cold shower. This is most people, as it is very uncommon to have just a bath with no shower available nowadays. This means that it is rather simple to just head into the bathroom and take a cold shower—something that has health benefits aplenty all on its own! Another benefit people experience when it comes to cold shower therapy is gradual exposure. As opposed to cold plunges, you can get into the shower with the water at a higher temperature, and then steadily lower that temperature to minimize discomfort. Also, cold showers have the ability to improve alertness, which is definitely helpful when paired with the other benefits mentioned.

On the other hand, there are a few drawbacks to be mindful of. Specifically, temperature control of a shower can be difficult to manage. A lot of people struggle to maintain consistent shower temperature throughout the duration of the shower, which is a very common struggle that can prove to be disadvantageous. Because of this, you can't really ensure that your showers are the same icy temperature each time without going to great lengths. Furthermore, not only does it take time for most people to get used to cold showers, but cold showers don't offer the full body immersion experience that most people crave when it comes to these methods. As a result, less benefits may be experienced.

So, as you can see, there are plenty of alternatives to cold plunges. These alternatives can benefit others but aren't for everyone. If you experience issues with traditional cold plunging, you might want to try those other methods I mentioned! To sum up the comparison:

- Temperature control. There are different temperature control aspects to keep in mind, and depending on how important this is to you, the clear winner is the cryotherapy chamber. Cold plunges tend to warm up too fast for some individuals, which is the result of body heat and ice coming into contact with one another. In addition, many showers struggle to maintain consistent temperature, and there's no way to

regulate a constant temperature across showers.
Because cryotherapy chambers are a bit more
extravagant, they naturally come with flawless
temperature controls that you can change to suit
your needs.

- Session duration. Depending on what you're
looking for when it comes to the duration of your
session, any option mentioned above can work for
you. The shortest option when it comes to
duration is the cryotherapy chamber, which is
often only used for two to three minutes at a time.
On the other hand, cold plunges can be used for
several more minutes, and cold showers can be
had for far more time than that still! So,
depending on what you particularly want when it
comes to your cold therapy sessions, you have the
ability to choose which method is going to benefit
your therapy based on duration.

- Convenience. For some people, convenience is the
make-or-break factor; other individuals don't
really care. This makes it vital to understand the
different convenience factors between the
available options. Cold showers are the easiest to
access; most people have a shower, and even if you
don't, public showers at gyms, pools, and even
saunas can provide a simple solution to that
matter. However, cryotherapy chambers are a lot
harder to come by. Cold plunges themselves fall in
between cold showers and cryotherapy chambers

on the convenience continuum, which makes them a good middle ground if you want more benefits than a shower but can't find the elusive cryotherapy chambers.

- Full body exposure. For a lot of people, the amount of bodily exposure during cold therapy is truly vital. For myself personally, I prefer methods that allow for full body immersion, and I know many individuals are the same way. If you're looking for full body exposure to the cold, then cold plunging or cryotherapy chambers are the way to go. While cold showers do have plenty of associated health benefits, they don't provide the same immersion experience as the other available options are able to.

- Potential health risks. One last aspect that is important to consider is the health risks that can be associated with these methods. If used improperly, a cryotherapy chamber can be dangerous or even deadly. On the opposite end of the scale, cold showers are usually completely safe, even if used daily or for a long duration. The implication of this is that prior to using a cryotherapy chamber or cold plunge, you should be aware of how to mitigate any potential health risks, as well as be aware that those health risks are possible in the first place.

Cold plunging can be a wonderful way to heal the body. Even on its own, cold plunging has a myriad of health benefits. And not only that, but it is quick and easy to build a cold plunge tub or pool right outside of your home, making cold plunging both simple and easy. Paired with the benefits of an indoor sauna—if you chose to design one for your home—your health is truly unstoppable! You have so many options for building the cold plunge of your dreams—and options if you don't want a cold plunge anyway.

Furthermore, keeping yourself safe is of the essence when it comes to cold plunging, and now you know how you can manage that as well. This chapter has truly empowered you to overcome some of the biggest struggles—and retain some of the most important knowledge—that comes along with cold plunging. In the next chapter, we will uncover everything you need to know about purchasing pre-made saunas and cold plunges alike, helping you achieve true success even if you are not handy around tools.

8

BUYING A PRE-MADE SAUNA AND COLD PLUNGE

H ow do I know which pre-made sauna or cold plunge kit is right for me? Buying the right kit can lead you to a wonderland of cold plunging and sauna experiences, but buying the wrong kit can be the grandest of disappointments. In Chapter 6, I mentioned how saunas can be installed from pre-packaged kits that contain everything you need; however, those kits alone can be a difficult maze to navigate. In order to success- fully find which premade option is right for you— avoiding a disaster in the process—you are going to need some guidance. That is what this chapter is all about.

EXPLORING PRE-MADE SAUNA AND COLD PLUNGE SYSTEMS

There is so much to know when it comes to pre-made sauna and cold plunge systems, but the good news is that I can break it all down for you. First thing's first, there are various pre-made sauna and cold plunge systems available, including traditional, infrared, and steam options. While not as authentic as building from scratch, these options are accessible for newcomers, making a compelling argument for starting here rather than constructing your own.

Pre-made Saunas

Let's start by talking about the pre-made sauna options that are available to you. Sauna kits come with everything you need in order to build or install your sauna from the ground up. There are various brands, types, and other options for pre-made sauna kits, even ones that customize the aesthetic of the experience. You can completely set these kits up on your own, which means that you do not need professionals or professional-grade tools to do so; in fact, most or all of the kits I've seen come with the tools in the box! How great is that? There are so many advantages that accompany the pre-made sauna kit as well, including (but certainly not limited to):

- Financially beneficial. Building a sauna to your specifications can cost upward of $5,000. Almost no one has that kind of cash lying around, and by going for lower-cost building materials, you also lower the quality of your sauna. However, buying a pre-made sauna kit can often be cheaper and more affordable, and the price truly does not mean lower quality! I've seen cheap and pre-made saunas that were far better than made-from-scratch saunas.

- Simple installation. Building a sauna from scratch can be confusing and overwhelming, especially if you are new to building and construction. However, pre-made kits come with everything you need and simplified instructions, which means that even someone who has never built a chair can manage a DIY pre-made sauna kit in just a few hours. This makes what could be a stressful experience become something that is sweet and simple.

- Easily maintained. Saunas that you make yourself are harder to keep up because of the fact that you personalize everything. On the other hand, pre-made saunas are organized with the expectation that you are a newbie (which there's no shame in). They come with maintenance instructions and can usually just be wiped down, which is a plus, and my favorite part is that these pre-made kits are usually covered by a warranty. This means that any damage is covered, sustaining the life of your sauna.

- Perfectly safe. Building your own sauna from scratch comes with a number of safety considerations, and by making a mistake in those considerations, you can put the life of yourself and others at risk; however, if you buy a pre-made kit, every safety issue is hammered out beforehand.

While there are a number of benefits to a pre-made sauna kit, there are also things that you have to consider before buying yours. For example, it is important to think about cost. The larger the sauna, the higher the cost, which makes sense as a bigger sauna is going to use more materials. Amenities, wood types, and other aspects also make a difference in the price, yet the overall price is still low for what you are getting. You also have to consider installation requirements, what wood you want, and more. All of this will be explored in depth in the final section of this chapter.

Pre-made Cold Plunges

In addition to pre-made saunas, you can purchase cold plunges in pre-arranged kits as well. While they are simple to build, the process can be further simplified by buying a ready-made cold plunge kit, including everything you need. In some instances, cold plunge kits even have most or all of the components assembled. Some aspects of a cold plunge kit that you should consider prior to buying include:

- Size. You can cold plunge alone or in a social environment, which means that you might opt to cold plunge with your family and/or friends. If you want a larger cold plunge to involve friends with, then that might up your cost, which is another consideration to make.

- Cost. Cold plunges and their materials are usually cheap, in fact much cheaper than a pre-made sauna kit would be. However, certain considerations like material, size, shape (yes, they come in really cool shapes), location, and more will impact the cost.
- Material. Do you want a cold plunge that is metal, plastic, or something else? Considering material is not just important from an aesthetic perspective; it is also important for ensuring that your cold plunge can retain the temperature of the water.
- Location. Whether you want your cold plunge to be situated in or out of doors matters as well. Not only does this impact size and shape, but outdoor cold plunges are going to be more durable. In addition, indoor cold plunges can damage your house if you are not careful about water levels, so consider whether that is a risk you are willing to take.

These options can be a great way to begin exploring the world of sauna and cold plunge therapies without extensive investment in time or craftsmanship. Whether you are not interested in building or just want to get to the benefits of saunas and cold plunges right away, ready-made kits can be an awesome option. Now, there might be a question lingering in your mind: Who do I buy my kit from? There are so many brands on the market that you might not know who to trust. Do not worry; I'll tell you!

RECOMMENDATIONS FOR RELIABLE BRANDS AND KEY FEATURES

Navigating the maze of sauna and cold plunge brands can be a challenge. There are hundreds of brands for each at the very least, and price alone cannot tell you which kits are going to be the best quality; instead, it is important to take a good look at some individual brands and features that will help you make the choice. The good news is that I know plenty of brands you might want to look into for your pre-made sauna and cold plunge needs.

Best Sauna Kits and Brands

Overall, if we consider all of the features and specifications of the available saunas, there's one that shines above all others. It is the Redwood Cedar Barrel Sauna. Holding up to six people, this beauty can be used as a dry sauna or a steam sauna effectively. It comes equipped with multiple different options for heaters and is even Wi-Fi compatible so that you can use your smartphone as a controller. That is just the greatest. Beyond that, this particular sauna can get up to ideal temperatures in under an hour. Quick and effective, this sauna is immensely spacious and comes with a vast number of optional add-ons that can enhance your experience. The drawbacks of this sauna are that the assembly can be a bit tricky, and it is one of the pricier options available.

If you are looking for a good in-home steam sauna, Renu Therapy's Rusticus sauna might be the perfect option. This sauna is the perfect size for couples or a group of three and is perfectly rust resistant. Made from domestically sourced wood, this beautiful steam sauna fits a rustic aesthetic and comes with versatile seating options. It can handle very high temperatures and parts of the sauna come pre-assembled, which is helpful for those not looking for a large construction project. This sauna also comes with temperature controls. On the downside, this sauna does require multiple people to move due to how heavy it is, which means that you should have someone help you when it arrives—that is, unless you want to unpackage and dismantle it on your porch.

They even sell kits for infrared saunas, as mentioned earlier. If this type of sauna is more your style, then the Luminar by Sun Home is a wonderful option. It can seat up to five people at once and the design is just beautiful. Made to last outside, this sauna also has magnetic locks that allow for simple assembly. It is one of the best for outdoor lighting and views and has full temperature diffusion throughout the interior. The sauna can be remotely controlled from a smartphone, and it has Bluetooth features as well as a lifetime warranty. If you do not mind the lack of a traditional experience, this sauna is perfect and certainly one of my favorites.

For a more traditional experience, I can safely recommend the Redwood Cedar Cube sauna. It comes with all of the quality and all of the specs of the Cedar Barrel mentioned earlier, but the seating is far more versatile and seats more people. Comfort is key with this sauna, and it even comes with many different heating options and Wi-Fi compatibility. You can plug it into a regular home outlet, and while assembly is going to be difficult with this sauna, yet again, keeping it outside is safe due to the quality of wood. You can even get upgraded roofing that prevents weather damage.

There are so many other types of saunas that I would recommend, but we would be here all day if I were to go into detail with each one. Some honorable mentions that are particularly worthwhile if you are not impressed already include:

- HigherDOSE Infrared Sauna Blanket. This sauna only fits one person, which makes sense; it is a blanket. You heard me right! HigherDOSE sells a sauna blanket that can allow you to achieve the same benefits as a normal sauna while... lying down under a blanket. Isn't that super cool? It is made of thick leather that protects your skin from the heating element. This blanket is huge but folds to a compact size and is portable for travel. While some users complain of the blanket taking a while to heat up or that the temperature controls were too vague, many enjoyed this convenient option for sauna usage.

- SweatTent Outdoor Sauna. This is yet another portable sauna option. Unlike the sauna blanket, this option can fit up to three people and can be left outside for good; however, it also makes a wonderful travel option. Heated by a wood power stove, your sauna also comes with rocks and everything you need for tending the fire. Dry heat allows you to relax without steam, although you can employ a steam method. One of my favorite parts about this option is that you can set it up (or tear it down) in under three minutes.
- Sun Home's Equinox. Another option by Sun Home is this wonderful infrared sauna. It can fit two people and is made entirely of pine, with hand-sanded wood for the highest quality around. This also comes with a modern Bluetooth speaker option and can be preheated, so no waiting is necessary. How nice!

With these sauna systems, the at-home sauna groove has never been smoother! You have the ability to have everything you need shipped right to your house, where you can safely assemble a quality sauna. Best of all, this purchase will not leave your pocket hurting afterward!

Best Cold Plunge Kits and Brands

Much like saunas, cold plunge kits can be purchased to make the process simpler. There are just as many cold plunge kits that you can find to suit your needs, including:

- Mueller Recovery Care Tub. One of the cheaper options available, this cold plunge kit can be used at home or packed up and taken with you on a trip. This can be a helpful tub if you are hoping to resolve injuries or even just have a relaxing dip in the ice. This tub is easy to set up and take down, and it is endorsed by athletic therapy specialists.
- Tru Grit Inflatable Ice Bath. Another cheap option, this tub is portable as well. Many people have mentioned not only that it works well with a standard hose, but that it is perfect for travel and flawless at keeping the water inside nice and cold. It is lightweight, and the biggest issue with this tub is that the brand lettering wears off fast—but who has a big problem with that anyway, am I right?
- Edge Theory Labs Edge Tub. This is a little pricier of an option, but financing is available if you are looking to buy it. One idiosyncratic benefit of this tub is that it comes with built in sanitation mechanisms, meaning that it works hard to stay clean so that you do not have to keep it clean. This tub is portable as well, but it is harder to set up

and take down, which may be a drawback for some.

- G Ganen Foldable Ice Bath. Cheap, portable, comfortable, and versatile—what more could one want from an ice bathtub? There are a few drawbacks of this tub—specifically that it can be hard to climb out of and that it has a bit of an odor at first—but overall, this option stands out for those looking for something simple and cheap to use for themselves.
- BlueCube Malibu 56 Cold Plunge. I'll be honest with you; this is an incredibly pricey option. Hear me out! Financing is available, and this is a quality tub that is good for both the home and a business. It has a chilling motor and is both energy efficient and low maintenance. It is self-contained, which means that you do not have to look at ugly wiring or hardware, and it is made built-to-order. This shipping wait time is totally worth it.
- Odin Ice Bath. Another pricier option, but in my opinion, it is totally worth it. You know why? This is the only ice bath/cold plunge tub on the market that makes its own ice! How impressive is that? It is also extremely easy to use, which is just another bonus to an already excellent tub. It can take a while to ship, and cleaning is a bit costly as well, but if you have the money to spend, this is 100% worth it.

Whether you opt to go with a sauna or cold plunge—or even both—you have so many options for pre-made kits that can make the building process far easier. All you need for these saunas is a little faith and the perfect spot picked out, and you are good to go. Before you click that order button, however, let's think about some practical considerations you might want to keep in mind for your first time purchasing one of these kits.

CONSIDERATIONS FOR THE FIRST-TIME BUYER

Before you buy your kit, it is important to keep a few considerations in mind; these considerations will ensure that your kit is perfectly suited for your needs, preventing costly returns or changes if it is not what you like. Instead of having to go through all of that, why not just start off with a tub you like? That sounds much better to me, so let's talk about some of the considerations you need to make in order to select the perfect sauna or cold plunge kit for you and your home.

Let's start with the elephant in the room: Cost. Perhaps one of the most important elements of getting a pre-made kit for a sauna or cold plunge is how much it is going to run you. It goes without saying that pre-made kits are cheaper than building a sauna or cold plunge yourself—at least in most cases—but that does not make the cost associated with pre-made kits anything less to consider. If you are on a budget, the typical price for a basic pre-made sauna kit is going to be around $2,000. This might sound like a lot, but keep in mind the fact that this includes *everything* you need, and it is several grand cheaper than making it from scratch. You can even find kits cheaper than that.

It is also important to consider the installation requirements of the kit you are planning to purchase. While everything you need comes in the kit already, you still have to think about a few things. For example, if you are setting up shop outside, then using a level surface is necessary. In other words, you cannot place your sauna or cold plunge on a sloped or bumpy surface. Doing so may cause it to malfunction, and even if the effects are not immediately apparent, you also risk permanently damaging the integrity of the sauna or plunge. A simple setup that is easy to move involves some wooden pallets and a tarp, but concrete or pavement works best.

Then, you have to choose the wood type if you are buying a sauna kit. For indoor saunas, the wood does not have to withstand the harsh elements of the outdoors; however, that is not the case for a sauna you operate outside. These saunas are going to need stronger wood that can handle moisture and mold alike, such as cedar, spruce, or pine. You should also ensure that you have the right permits if your sauna is going outside, as technically a sauna is considered a building and, therefore, needs special permits. Besides, who wants a ticket or legal troubles from a sauna?

Buying your very own sauna kit for the first time is not the easiest thing in the world, unless you have the right guide that is. Luckily for you, you have just finished reading about all of the different aspects of buying a sauna kit. Not only do you know the advantages of doing so, but you know what brands to look for as well as what considerations need to be made in order to ensure that your first kit is a success. Right on!

9

INCORPORATING SAUNA AND COLD PLUNGE INTO YOUR LIFESTYLE

Your sauna and cold plunge journey is not complete. You do not have to make your life about sauna and cold plunge usage. After all, your life was never about brushing your teeth in the morning, now, was it? However, brushing your teeth is a valuable part of your overall lifestyle that invites health and wellness into your life, and this is exactly what you should aim to do with saunas and cold plunging. When you integrate these health aspects into your overall lifestyle, then you have the increased ability to maintain health and wellness entirely and holistically. So, let's begin learning how to integrate saunas and cold plunge into your lifestyle overall.

INTEGRATING SAUNA AND COLD PLUNGE INTO DAILY OR WEEKLY ROUTINES

You're busy, I get it. I know better than anyone else just how busy life can be. Unfortunately, this means that you might not have the ability to cold plunge or use a sauna on a daily basis, which is understandable and not necessary to achieve stellar benefits. Whether you plan to integrate cold plunge and sauna into a daily routine or just a weekly one, you have the power to integrate these healthy habits into your routine as a part of your overall lifestyle.

Let's start with some numbers. It is best to get in at least 12 minutes of cold therapy and an hour of heat therapy a week. You can divide this however you want. For example, you can get in your cold therapy in two six-minute sessions during a nice Saturday, or you can go for two minutes a day every day. Either way, you are reaping the same health benefits. The same goes for heat therapy.

Now, it is time to think about when to put your heat and cold therapy into your schedule. If you are going to do so once a week, then I suggest doing so at the very start of your week, giving you an energetic physical and mental boost. On the other hand, if you plan to engage with these habits on a daily basis, then it is best to do so at the beginning of the day. This allows you to carry those benefits throughout the day. You should also aim to start with a cold plunge, then hit the sauna, and finally, finish off with the cold plunge again. This employs the benefits of contrast therapy for the greatest benefits.

Starting off with implementing all of these changes can be a bit much. This is why it is important to slowly build up your routine. Whether you are going for once a week or once a day as your goal, or even multiple times a day, starting off slow with shorter periods of time can build up the consistency that is necessary for a habit to be advantageous. For example, if you cannot get 12 minutes of cold during the course of a week, then you can go for two minutes a week at first; let your body get used to the routine.

In order for habits to stick, it is said to take three weeks. Over the course of the three weeks that you plan to engage with this habit, make sure to engage at the same time and day (or days) every week for the best impact. By doing so, your brain comes to understand that, for instance, 2 p.m. on Sunday is cold plunge time. This connects your brain and the habit together intimately.

A PATH TO WELLNESS: EMBRACING HEAT AND COLD

Saunas and cold plunges alike boost the level of dopamine in your brain. What does that even mean? Well, allow me to explain! Dopamine is the chemical in your brain that is, in many ways, responsible for happiness and pleasure. If we do not have enough dopamine in the brain, it can result in depression, anxiety, and other mental health conditions. As it turns out, one of the ways that you can boost dopamine is to put stress on the body. For example, exercise is often considered to be one of the best ways to boost dopamine levels. The body does this because it thinks you will be in pain, and therefore sends out dopamine to prevent that pain.

When you engage with a sauna or a cold plunge, you also boost your dopamine in a similar way; it makes your body think you are in harm's way or otherwise very uncomfortable, and as a result, it forces your body to release dopamine. This makes you feel pleasure and comfort when you engage with a sauna or cold plunge rather than the discomfort that may be associated with these experiences when you think about them.

In fact, this is why cold plunges and saunas can even feel addictive—in a positive way, of course. The more you visit a sauna or a cold plunge, the more you will crave the experience in order to attain the positive benefits and the dopamine boosts that it can cause. This is a way that the positive habit is reinforced in the mind, keeping us on track with our positive habits and goals. In a way, you become addicted to the good feeling, and it is not dangerous to love health!

Other Practices for Wellness

Did you know that there are other wellness practices that can enhance the benefits of saunas and cold plunge experiences? Namely, yoga and meditation can make the experience more beneficial from a holistic standpoint, helping you feel better mentally, physically, and even spiritually.

If you remember, I mentioned earlier that a bigger sauna is good for those who plan to do yoga while in the sauna. This form of yoga, commonly referred to as hot yoga, is beneficial due to the paired benefits of yoga and using a sauna. But you do not have to do yoga inside of the sauna to reap the positive benefits. As mentioned earlier, saunas work great before and/or after a workout depending on your goals, and if you want to do yoga inside of the sauna, you totally can—provided that you have space.

Meditation also goes particularly well with a sauna. One advantage of this practice paired with a sauna or cold plunge is that you can practice mindfulness in the sauna or cold plunge without much additional effort. Not only does mindfulness take your mind off of any physical discomfort that you might be feeling, but it also helps clear your mind, raise awareness, and has even been linked to decreased depression and anxiety. Forming a mindfulness practice for while you are inside the sauna or cold plunge is so beneficial!

NUTRITION AND HYDRATION FOR SAUNAS AND COLD PLUNGING

Proper nutrition and hydration are vital for someone who expects health benefits from a sauna or cold plunge. For many people, this is something that can necessitate a handful of lifestyle changes; after all, not everyone is immediately aware of the effects that nutrition and hydration can have on health and thus sauna or cold plunge usage. Therefore, we need to talk about it!

On Hydration, Saunas, and Cold Plunging

For saunas especially, hydration is something you cannot ignore. Because saunas make you sweat so much, you lose fluids that your body needs. This puts you at severe risk of dehydration if you do not stay hydrated. One aspect of hydration that is important to take note of is a proper fluid balance. Due to the fact that saunas can make you lose so much fluid through the heat you are exposed to, you can be at risk of losing your body's natural fluid balance. Signs of dehydration that you should look out for include dizziness, muscle cramps, and heat stroke. This is one of the reasons why it is important to never lock yourself inside of a sauna.

Making sure that you are properly hydrated is not just important for that reason either. Something else that proper hydration does is ensure that your body experiences proper thermoregulation. In other words, drinking enough water and remaining hydrated helps your body regulate its temperature more effectively. Immediately, this might sound like the antithesis of what you want; should your body temperature regulation being low not help the effects? And the answer is "no." When you have proper temperature regulation, you can withstand the extreme temperatures longer, thus achieving more benefits. It is not about being miserable; that is not what gives you the benefits!

In addition, hydration is important because it improves circulation. This is because when you are dehydrated, your blood becomes thicker. It is true! If you have ever seen someone pinch the back of someone else's hand to test for dehydration, what they're testing for is to see if the skin snaps back into place; if not, that person is very dehydrated and, therefore, their blood is thicker. This also means that they're suffering from poor circulation. Maintaining good circulation is essential for saunas and cold plunging to have the benefits you expect; a lot of the benefits that we talked about are due to circulation, after all.

Finally, hydration is important for muscle function. One of the most common reasons that people endure saunas or cold plunging is because they can benefit the process of muscle repair; that is no good if you do not actually take the proper steps to help your body experience said muscular benefits. When you are dehydrated, your muscles cannot stretch or flex as well. In fact, they actively start to cramp. This can damage the muscle tissue more, especially if you get into a sauna that further dehydrates you! Because of this, drinking enough water during workouts and sauna usage is of the essence.

As you can see, it is crucial that you ensure good hydration and nutrition practices in order to get the most out of your sauna and/or cold plunge experience; by neglecting your hydration and nutrition, you do not just risk losing out on benefits—you also risk your life, and that is not a joke.

On Nutrition, Saunas, and Cold Plunging

There are many reasons that nutrition is important for saunas and cold plunging as well. If you are engaging with these activities to support weight loss, you might think that nutrient deprivation is not all that bad—and you are wrong. Let's talk about why that is.

One of the reasons that nutrition is so important for sauna and cold plunge usage is that nutrition contributes massively to the body's energy supply. The foods you eat play a major role in how much energy you have. Carbohydrates, for example, serve as the body's primary food source for energy. When you enter a sauna or cold plunge, your body fights to be able to regulate and maintain its temperature. This process is important because it is what keeps you from literal death when you submerge yourself in these temperatures. In order to do so, however, your body must expend energy. This means that consuming a snack or balanced meal prior to hopping in the sauna or cold plunge (waiting at least a half-hour in between) can actually help your body attain health benefits more productively.

Furthermore, because the process of participating in a sauna or cold plunge can be rather strenuous on the body, your body might actually need recovery from the sauna or cold plunge itself so that you can sustain the benefits. This is another component wherein nutrition can be beneficial! Consuming nutrients *after* a sauna or cold plunge experience can do wonders for the recovery process. Specifically, protein and carbohydrate-rich foods can aid in replenishing energy and glycogen stores, both of which can then ensure that your muscles and organs sustain no harm from the harsh temperatures you endured.

Electrolytes are also important to think about. After an athlete plays a game of sports, you can frequently see them drinking Gatorade or another electrolyte drink. This is because sweating depletes your electrolyte stores, therefore dehydrating you, as your body tries to keep itself cool in an otherwise very warm environment. The sweating that you do as a result of sauna usage—and sometimes as a result of cold plunge usage—similarly depletes your body of electrolytes. Specifically, you might find yourself lacking in the essential electrolytes of sodium, potassium, and magnesium. Therefore, consuming foods that are rich in these minerals can support muscle health and fluid balance for overall improvement in your well-being.

Lastly, it is important to consider the impact that antioxidant and anti-inflammatory foods can have on your experience with saunas and cold plunging. Extreme temperatures like cold and hot can lower inflammation, but in some individuals, they actually cause it. For those instances, anti-inflammatory foods can be a game changer. Likewise, for those who experience oxidative stress as a result of sauna or cold plunge usage, antioxidant foods can be particularly beneficial.

So, as you can see, nutrition is equally as important as hydration when it comes to using the sauna or cold plunge methods for health. But what can be done to minimize risks and ensure proper usage of saunas and cold plunges with this in mind?

Minimizing Risk With Lifestyle Changes

Certain lifestyle changes that are simple, yet impactful, can truly make a difference when it comes to minimizing any hazards that are associated with saunas. When you do not eat or drink enough, your body is not quite sure how to interpret external stimuli. As a result, it might respond to heat or cold far differently, and that is not a good thing. Because of this, it is important to maintain proper nutrition and hydration in order to allow your body to interpret temperature well; this means that your body will send proper cues for when it is time to get out of the cold plunge or sauna. This can prevent dangerous overindulgence. Moreover, taking the time to make these changes can prevent fainting, overheating, and more.

SAUNA AND COLD PLUNGE SAFETY FOR CHILDREN AND SENIORS

Implementing saunas and cold plunging into the lives of seniors and children might seem like a good idea, and in moderation it can definitely serve one well. However, there are also safety considerations that need to be kept in mind due to the unique vulnerabilities of each group. For example, some safety considerations that you need to keep in mind for children include:

- Age and maturity level. Depending on the age and maturity of a given child, they may or may not be able to handle sauna or cold plunge therapy. Younger children tend to have a lower tolerance for extreme temperatures, and this is not because they're stubborn! Younger children genuinely have a lesser ability to regulate their body temperature, which can contribute to cold or heat being not only immensely uncomfortable but actually dangerous. As such, knowing your child specifically as well as their limits and maturity is important to think about. Generally, it is not recommended to introduce children under 12 to saunas or cold plunges.
- Supervision. So, you have an older child who you want to introduce to the wonderful world of saunas or cold plunging; that is excellent! However, you cannot just toss them into the

experience and leave them to it. Children who engage in sauna or cold plunge experiences should always be monitored closely by an adult. They should also be aware of safety guidelines and be able to communicate distress (and that communication should be respected). Furthermore, as a parent, it is part of your job to be on the lookout for obvious signs of discomfort or distress that indicate that your child should be removed from the sauna or cold plunge. Remember, this impacts their health and life, so do not play around!

- Time limits. Adults can typically handle longer periods of time in the sauna, but just as you have to gradually work up to that increased time, so does your child. However, even a short 15-minute session can be too much for a small child, so try going for an even shorter session of just five minutes. Not only does this help them become acquainted with the sensations of a sauna, but it teaches their body that they're safe and can relax within such a pressurized circumstance. Over time, you can gradually introduce your child to longer sessions until they become comfortable with it. This also goes for cold plunging!

- Hydration. Just as it is important for adults to be hydrated both before and after the usage of a sauna, it is important for children to do so as well. If you plan on introducing your child to a sauna, make sure that they drink plenty of water both before and after the experience. If you explain to your child how this can help and why this is important, not only will it become a learning experience, but they will likely be far more willing to participate.

- Cooling down. Even for adults, taking the time to cool down or warm up after a sauna experience is vital. This makes it just as important for children. After your child exits the experience, allow them to sit in a comfortable environment with a cup of water and just relax. Let them do this for at least 30 minutes; even if they say they feel fine, do not let them run around or exert themselves, as this can be harmful, and children often do not know their bodies very well yet.

- Health conditions. Children have far more sensitive bodies than adults, and that sensitivity is heightened for children with pre-existing health conditions. If your child has a health condition, such as a heart problem or respiratory issue, then you should avoid saunas or cold plunging unless specifically directed otherwise by a medical professional. No health benefits are worth risking your child's life.

On a more personal note, I truly recommend not forcing your child into a cold plunge or sauna; they will have a more enjoyable experience if you get them excited for it and treat it like a fun experience rather than one of force.

Seniors also have specific requirements for safety that should be considered, including:

- Healthcare consultation. Seniors should always make sure to speak to a healthcare professional before implementing any major changes into their lifestyle, and saunas and cold plunging are no different. There are many reasons why doing so is a good idea, and you really should not skip out on this aspect. If you have heart or lung problems, take medication, or experience a health condition that impacts blood pressure, alertness, or temperature regulation, then you should be extra careful to consider a healthcare professional's advice before partaking in a sauna or cold plunge experience; otherwise, you risk experiencing damaging health impacts that outweigh any potential benefits.
- Medication awareness. As mentioned in the last point, certain medications put one at a higher risk of complications when combined with the severe temperature pressures of a sauna or cold plunge. Because of this, it is important to be aware of the impacts that some medication can have, especially if you do take any medication. Before jumping in the sauna or cold plunging, thoroughly research

how your medication impacts your temperature control and/or blood pressure. Furthermore, certain medications can make you more susceptible to temperature-related illness as well as dehydration. If you are confused or concerned —I know I would be—reach out to your doctor. They can provide you with more specific guidance than I could!

- Neutral temperatures and shorter sessions. Those who are older should opt for more neutral temperatures that are closer to their body temperature; for instance, saunas should be cooler and cold plunges should be warmer than the usual temperature. Furthermore, sessions should be shorter than an adult in the early stages of their life would go for. This can help seniors adapt to the temperatures more gradually as well as avoid complications due to the extreme temperatures. I recommend starting off with a safe, comfortable temperature and then slowly increasing or decreasing the temperature, depending on what you are doing.

- Moderation. When it comes to both the duration and frequency of sauna and cold plunge sessions, seniors have to be especially careful. While it is possible for younger individuals to go for a sauna or cold plunge experience every single day, seniors definitely shouldn't aim for this. Exposing oneself to extreme temperatures, especially as you reach older ages, can put certain and severe strain on the cardiovascular system, which means putting unnecessary strain on the heart. Especially if one has an underlying heart condition, overexposure to saunas or cold plunging can have dire side effects.

- Hydration. Hydration is important for everyone when taking advantage of the benefits associated with saunas and cold plunging, but it is especially important for seniors. One thing that is important to note is that the older you become, the more your thirst perception changes. This means that you might not know that you need water when you're severely dehydrated. As a result, it is a good idea to drink plenty of water before and after a sauna or cold plunge experience because this reduces the risk you face of suffering from dehydration or overheating. So, even if you don't *feel* thirsty, make sure to drink plenty of water.

- Listen to your body. As you get older, your body changes in a plethora of ways. Sometimes, this can prompt you to ignore the signals that your body is giving you, underestimating just how important they can be. This is never a good idea when it comes to something like saunas and cold plunging. If your body is providing you with signs that the sauna or cold plunge is too much, always listen to those signals; otherwise, you could face serious injury or health issues. Some signs that you should take note of include feeling lightheaded, dizzy, or unwell. If the feelings persist after exiting, be sure to seek immediate assistance, as you might be experiencing a medical emergency.

- Accessibility. Accessibility is always important, but for seniors it is of the essence. Due to the fact that many seniors experience balance and mobility issues, keeping accessibility features in mind is important. A senior-accessible sauna will have safety rails and bars, non-slip features, and more to ensure that no one is injured. Cold plunge tubs should be easy to get in and out of as well.

You truly cannot expect to maintain flawless health and wellness if you do not integrate sauna and cold plunge usage into your lifestyle as a whole. If you simply make it a thing you do sometimes when you feel like it, then the habit will not stick; just like brushing your teeth, consistency and habit are what matter most. Now, you have the empowering ability to integrate both saunas and cold plunging into your lifestyle. Next, we can take a look at scientific studies, case studies, and testimonials in support of saunas and cold plunging, finalizing the benefits and knowledge of your journey.

10

CELEBRITY TESTIMONIALS, SUCCESS STORIES, AND CASE STUDIES

I f you have not been convinced, or if you are purely curious about just how much others love these methods, then this chapter is for you. Believe it or not, success stories and case studies are so important to me; they lay the foundation for how I retain and trust knowledge because I believe that first-hand experience is far more telling than just what we know in our minds. With case studies and evidence, we push ourselves to meet our goals and achieve greatness. This chapter centers around the experiences that others have had with saunas and cold plunges and the success that they've experienced. Hopefully, this chapter inspires you to become a success story of your very own!

CELEBRITY TESTIMONIALS

As it turns out, hundreds of celebrities can attest to the benefits of saunas and cold plunges alike. One example of a celebrity who stands behind the benefits of saunas is Gwyneth Paltrow. Paltrow is a fan of health and wellness; thus, it makes perfect sense that she takes advantage of the benefits of saunas. She is known to use an infrared sauna as her sauna of choice, and she tries to stay inside of the sauna as much as she healthily can. Her day involves a regular routine of sauna usage, and she says that it makes her feel and look so much better. If you were ever wondering what her secret was, now you know!

Selena Gomez is another celebrity who is in love with saunas, specifically the infrared sauna. In one interview, Gomez mentioned that she's not one to work out very intensely. As a result, she opts for sauna usage instead. She says this makes her skin glow, keeps her in good shape, and makes her feel so much better. Gomez even attests to using an infrared sauna blanket, so if you were wondering whether that sauna blanket I mentioned earlier really works, it totally does!

In addition, Lady Gaga uses saunas as well. If you did not know, Lady Gaga has fibromyalgia, which is a chronic condition associated with many effects. Among the most harrowing involves chronic pain, and if you have ever experienced chronic pain, then you know it is no joke. Gaga has mentioned before that the use of an infrared sauna is particularly helpful when it comes to alleviating pain and reducing the symptoms of a flare up. She uses hers every single day for the best benefits.

And that is not even scratching the surface of the celebrities who use saunas. Cold plunges are also popular among celebrities, with those who use them including:

- Kevin Hart. A celebrity and comedian, Hart actually has a whole talk show dedicated to interviewing others while sitting in an ice bath. This is both because he loves how it feels and because it can help the body recover from the woes of intense physical activity.
- Chris Hemsworth. When Hemsworth filmed Thor, he had to engage in various strenuous workouts to fit the role. As a result, he experienced different results, including some of the hardships that accompany exercise like muscle and joint issues. Due to his personal trainer's guidance, Hemsworth meticulously plans when he intends to cold plunge, using it as a method to drastically improve muscle repair.
- Harry Styles. Styles is actually known for his love of cold plunging and swimming in cold water. This is part of the routine for how he recovers after a concert or other performance, and he says that it helps him remain physically and mentally well enough to continue touring.

Wow! That is a lot of people who notably care about their health and take advantage of saunas and cold plunges.

SUCCESS STORIES: REAL PEOPLE, REAL RESULTS

You do not have to be a celebrity to enjoy the benefits of saunas and cold plunges; ordinary people just like me and you can experience the same benefits and include these practices into our routines the exact same way.

For example, Jennifer Davis-Flynn of Yoga Journal had incredible experiences after using an infrared sauna for 30 consecutive days. Being candidly honest, Davis-Flynn said that the sauna did not change her life like many people claim; however, it definitely was an experience accompanied by unique health benefits and advantages, making it worthwhile for those seeking those particular benefits. She also mentioned that infrared saunas feel more authentic to a modern experience, whereas traditional saunas might not provide that same feel.

SCIENTIFIC STUDIES: DOCTORS' CASE STUDIES AND ENDORSEMENTS

Finally, let's focus on some scientific studies and endorsements of sauna and cold plunge usage. There are perhaps thousands of endorsements from doctors and professionals alike. Some of my favorites include:

- One study concluded that dry heat saunas have health benefits and did not indicate any significant health disadvantages that arise as a result of sauna usage (Hussain & Cohen, 2018).
- Another study concluded that benefits to the cardiovascular system could be appreciated, such as the lowering of blood pressure, as well as that there are health benefits like the decrease of headaches, arthritis, and the flu that result from regular sauna usage (Laukkanen et al., 2018).

Now that you have seen how others are impacted by saunas and cold plunges, why not make the success story your own? It is time to embark upon your journey at last, implementing everything you have learned over the last 10 chapters.

CONCLUSION

Throughout this journey, you have come to understand so much about hot and cold therapy through the power of saunas and cold plunges, which are the two keys to unlock magnified health. Now, you can truly drive your own journey into wellness without relying so much on other methods to guide you; instead, you can let the simple heat and cold benefit your health.

Whether you are building everything yourself or buying a pre-made kit, there are dozens of benefits to be enjoyed. From lowering inflammation to improving muscle health and more, the benefits associated with these two practices are unlike anything else I've ever discovered. I'm so grateful that I've had the opportunity to share what I know with you. If you have found this book to be beneficial, consider leaving a review so that others have access to this invaluable information.

The path to a healthier, happier life through sauna and cold plunge therapies is yours to explore. Start your journey today by embracing these age-old practices, knowing that you have all the tools, insights, and inspiration right here in your hands.

REFERENCES

3 Benefits of Sauna to Improve Your Yoga Practice. (n.d.). Sauna House. Retrieved September 10, 2023, from https://www.saunahouse.com/ blogs/wellness-guide/3-benefits-of-sauna-to-improve-your-yoga-practice#:~:text=When%20you%20decide%20to%20go

5 Interesting Facts about Sauna Use. (n.d.). Prairie Naturopathic Doctors. Retrieved September 9, 2023, from https://prairiend.com/blog/5-interesting-facts-about-sauna-use

8 Ice Bath Dos and Dont's | Urban Ice Tribe. (2022, July 11). https://urban icetribe.com/8-ice-bath-dos-and-donts/

11 Best Cold Plunge Tubs of 2023. (2023, June 30). Healthline. https://www. healthline.com/health/best-cold-plunge-tubs#comparison

13 Proven Ways Saunas Can Improve Your Mental Health. (n.d.). Optimal Living Dynamics. https://www.optimallivingdynamics.com/blog/ 13-proven-ways-saunas-can-improve-your-mental-health-dry-hot-benefits-depression-anxiety

19 Celebrities That Use a Cold Plunge As Part Of Their Wellness Routine - My Seven Chakras. (2023, January 22). My Seven Chakras. https://mysev enchakras.com/celebrities-that-use-a-cold-plunge

Adam. (2023, January 22). *10 Celebrities Who Love the Sauna*. TheSauna-Guide. https://thesaunaguide.com/10-cclcbrities-who-love-the-sauna/

Andonian, N. (2022, August 19). *The 13 Sauna Benefits for Your Health and Body*. GoodRx; GoodRx. https://www.goodrx.com/well-being/alter native-treatments/sauna-benefits

Beker, B. M. (2018). Human Physiology in Extreme Heat and Cold. *Clin-medjournals.org, 1*(1). https://doi.org/10.23937/iacph-2017/1710001

Dennison, A. (2023, March 2). *DIY Cold Plunge: 6 of the Best Do-It-Yourself Ice Bath Options -*. Coldplungefacts.com. https://coldplungefacts. com/diy-cold-plunge-6-best-options/#DIY_Cold_Plunge_Tub

Dunnett, T. (2022, February 12). *7 Different Types of Saunas Explained*. Sauna Samurai. https://www.saunasamurai.com/types-of-saunas/

Gibson, O. R., Taylor, L., Watt, P. W., & Maxwell, N. S. (2017). Cross-Adaptation: Heat and Cold Adaptation to Improve Physiological and Cellular Responses to Hypoxia. *Sports Medicine, 47*(9), 1751–1768. https://doi.org/10.1007/s40279-017-0717-z

Health and safety considerations. (2015, January 7). https://www.tylolife.co.uk/sauna-bathing/enjoying-your-sauna/health-and-safety-considerations/#:~: text=Building%20or%20designing%20a%20safe%20sauna.&text =All%20sauna%20doors%20should%20open%20outwards%20-for%20safety%20reasons.&text=The%20sauna%20-door%20should%20not

Higgins, S. (2022, October 17). *Contrast Therapy: All The Health Benefits You Need to Know.* HANA. https://hana.nz/journal/contrast-therapy-all-the-health-benefits-you-need-to-know/#:~:text=Finally%2C%20-contrast%20therapy%20aids%20natural

Hormesis - an overview | ScienceDirect Topics. (n.d.). Www.sciencedirect.com. https://www.sciencedirect.com/topics/agricultural-and-biological-sciences/hormesis#:~:text=Hormesis%20is%20defined%20as%20a

How Ice Baths Can Improve Your Mental Health. (2022, June 13). Plunge. https://plunge.com/en-ca/blogs/blog/how-ice-baths-can-improve-your-mental-health

Hussain, J., & Cohen, M. (2018). Clinical Effects of Regular Dry Sauna Bathing: A Systematic Review. *Evidence-Based Complementary and Alternative Medicine, 2018,* 1–30. https://doi.org/10.1155/2018/1857413

Laukkanen, J. A., Laukkanen, T., & Kunutsor, S. K. (2018). Cardiovascular and Other Health Benefits of Sauna Bathing: A Review of the Evidence. *Mayo Clinic Proceedings, 93*(8), 1111–1121. https://doi.org/10.1016/j.mayocp.2018.04.008

Marketplace, S. (2023, September 4). *This Sauna and Cold Plunge Routine Will Change Your Life.* https://saunamarketplace.com/sauna-cold-plunge-routine/

Potential Cold-Water Therapy and Ice Bath Benefits. (n.d.). EverydayHealth.com. https://www.everydayhealth.com/wellness/possible-health-benefits-to-cold-water-therapy/

PREFAB SAUNA: THE PERFECT BLEND OF COMFORT AND CONVE-

NIENCE. (n.d.). My Sauna World. Retrieved September 15, 2023, from https://mysaunaworld.com/blogs/my-sauna-world-blog/conve nience-and-comfort-of-a-prefab-sauna

Sauna: Health benefits, risks, and precautions. (n.d.). Www.medicalnewsto-day.com. https://www.medicalnewstoday.com/articles/313109#what-is-a-sauna

Saunas, C. I. (2019, March 21). *How to Build a Sauna: DIY Infrared Sauna Tips*. Clearlight Infrared Saunas. https://infraredsauna.com/blog/how-to-build-a-sauna-diy-infrared-sauna-tips/

Self Build Sauna Instructions | Finnmark Sauna Do it Yourself. (n.d.). Finnmark Sauna. Retrieved September 12, 2023, from https://finnmark sauna.com/en-us/blogs/sauna-how-to-guides/self-build-sauna-instructions

Team, S. org. (2018, December 1). *The History of Saunas*. Saunas.org. https://saunas.org/the-history-of-saunas/

The 7 Best Home Saunas of 2023 - Sports Illustrated. (n.d.). *Sports Illustrated*. Retrieved September 15, 2023, from https://www.si.com/showcase/fitness/best-home-sauna

TYPES OF SAUNAS: A COMPREHENSIVE GUIDE TO FINDING THE IDEAL SAUNA. (n.d.). My Sauna World. Retrieved September 12, 2023, from https://mysaunaworld.com/blogs/my-sauna-world-blog/different-types-of-saunas

What Is a Contrast Bath? (n.d.). WebMD. https://www.webmd.com/pain-management/what-is-a-contrast-bath

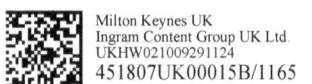